Esophagitis and Gastritis - Recent Updates

Edited by Vincenzo Neri and Monjur Ahmed

Published in London, United Kingdom

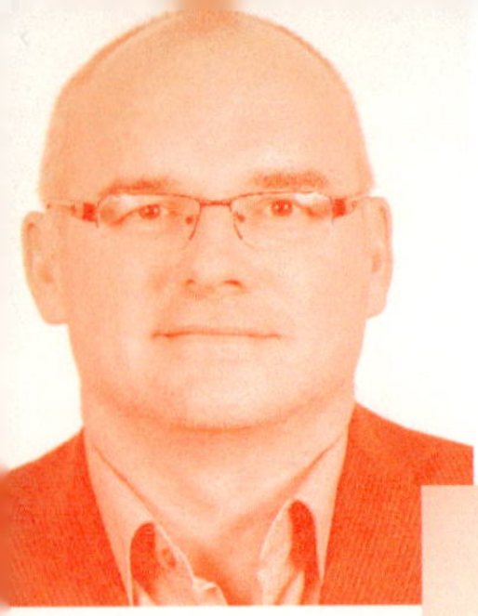
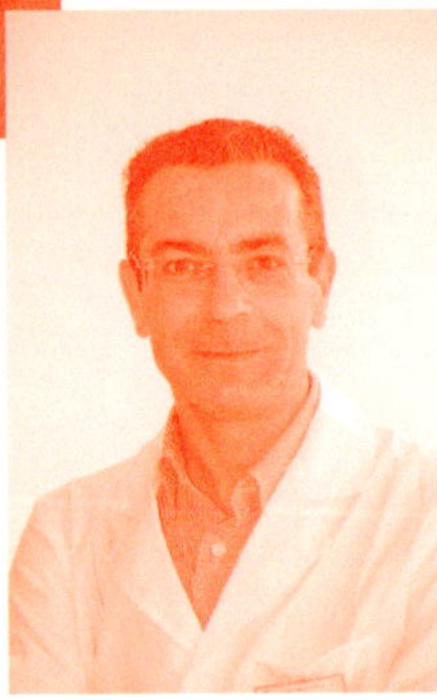
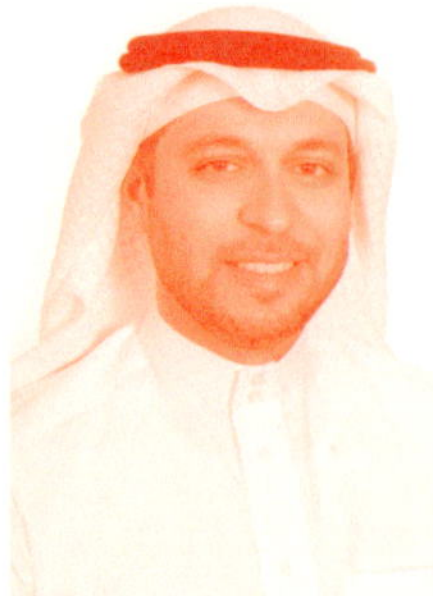
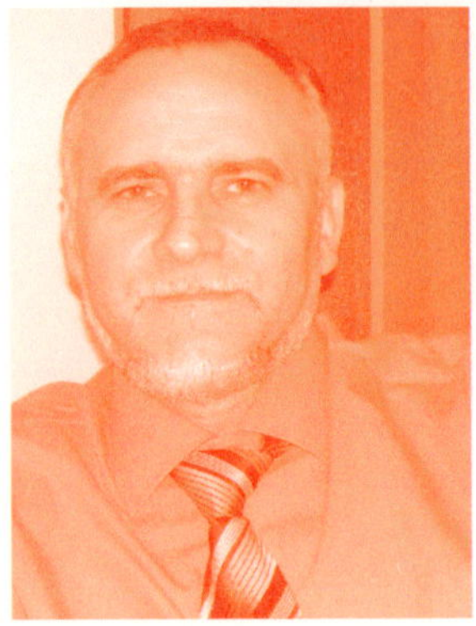
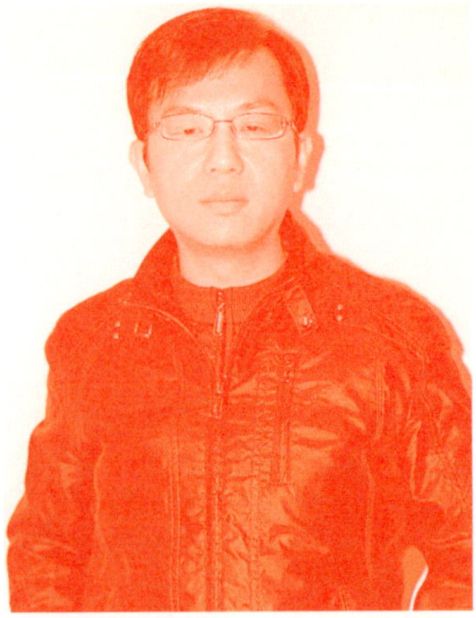
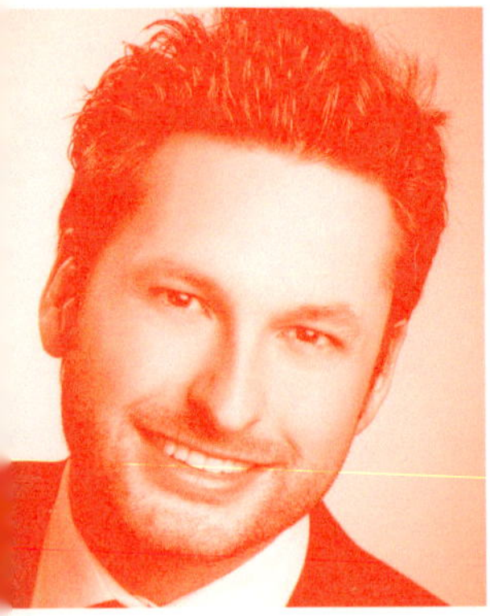
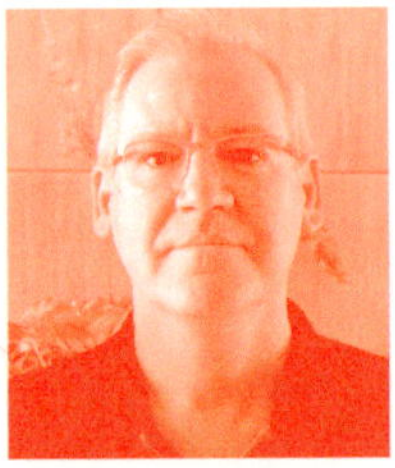

IntechOpen

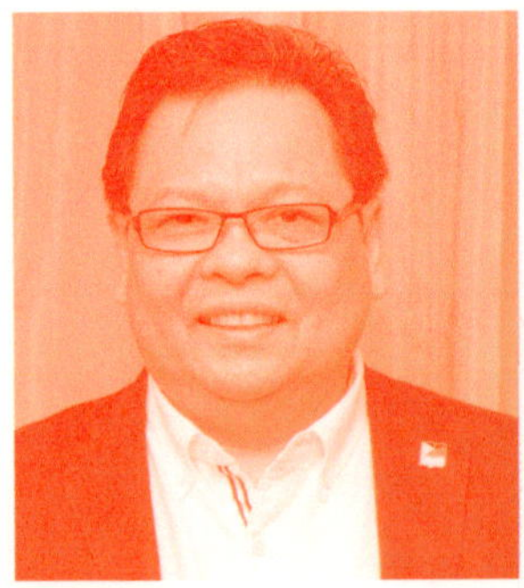
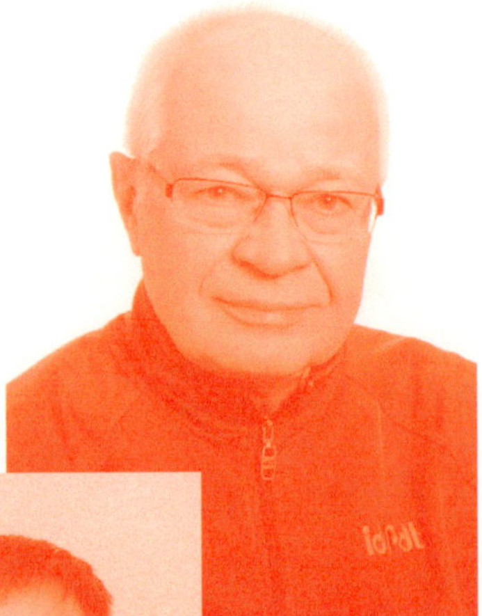
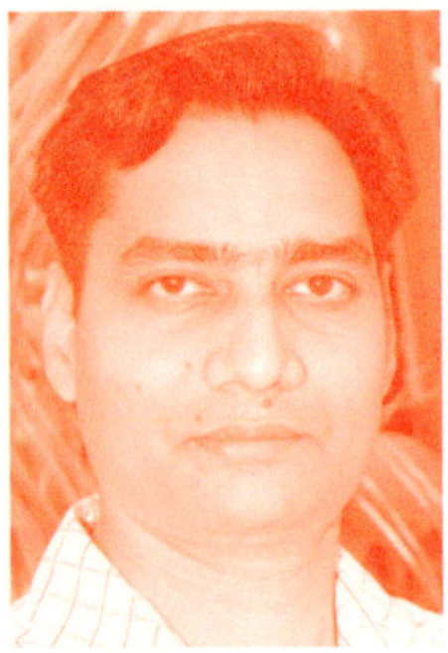
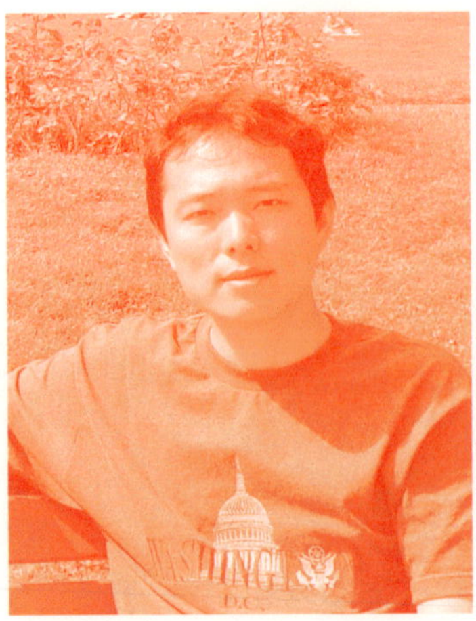
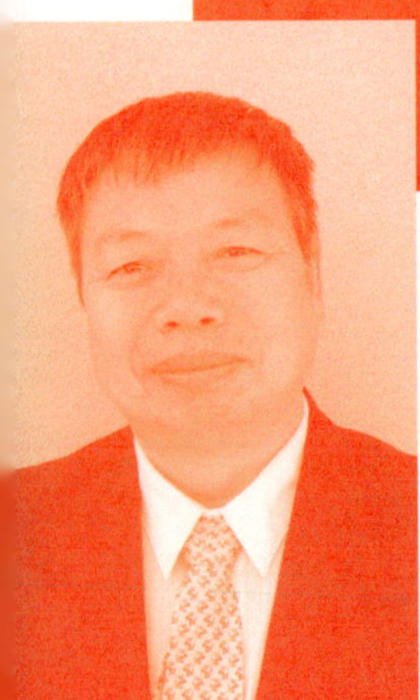
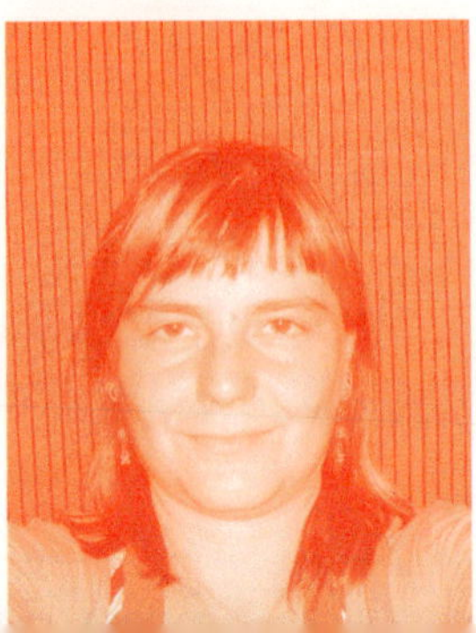

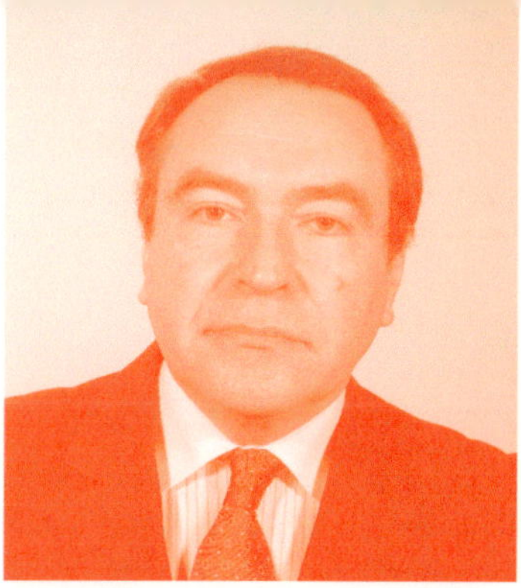
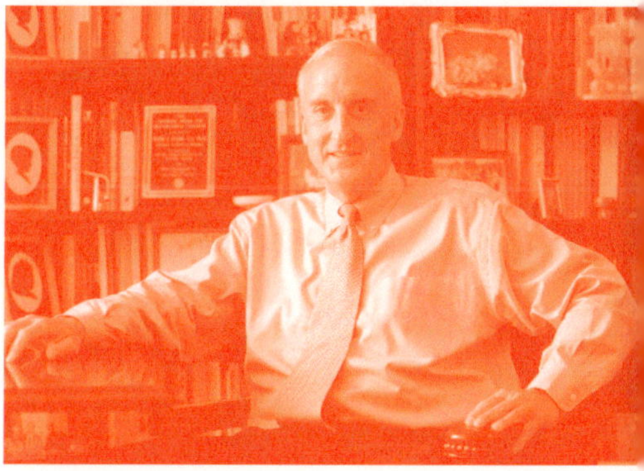
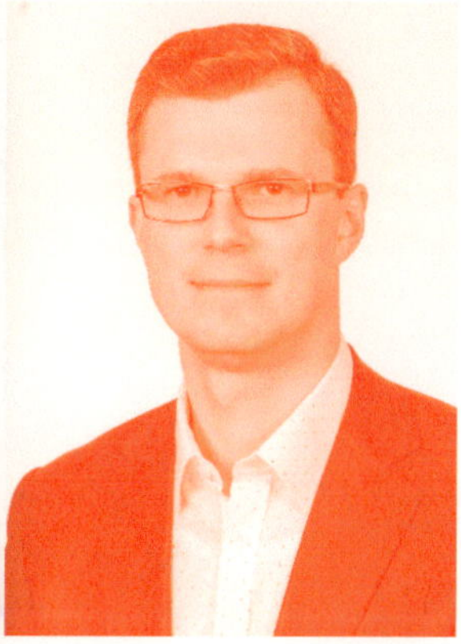
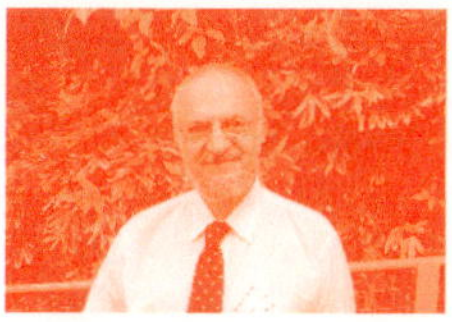
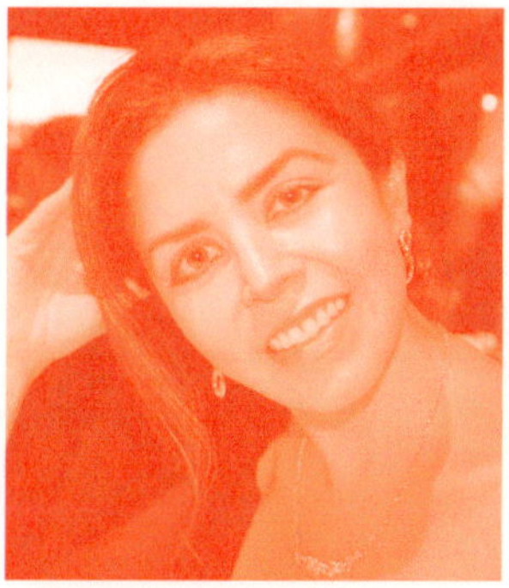

Supporting open minds since 2005

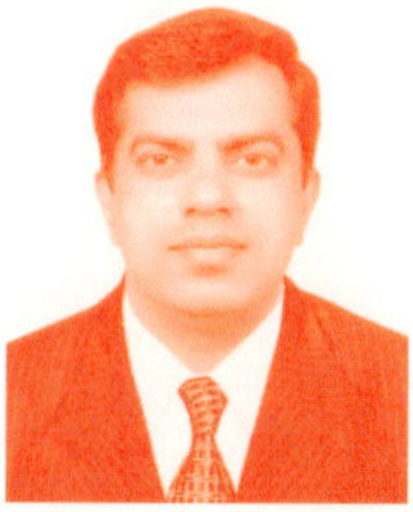
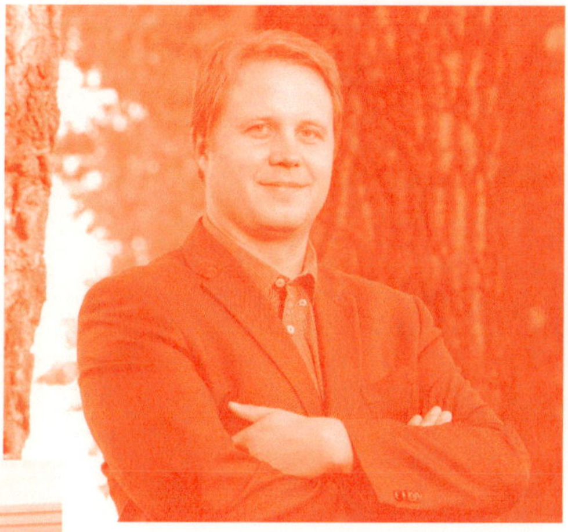
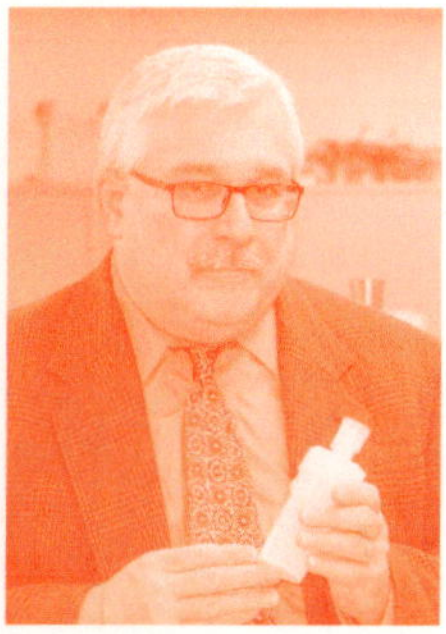
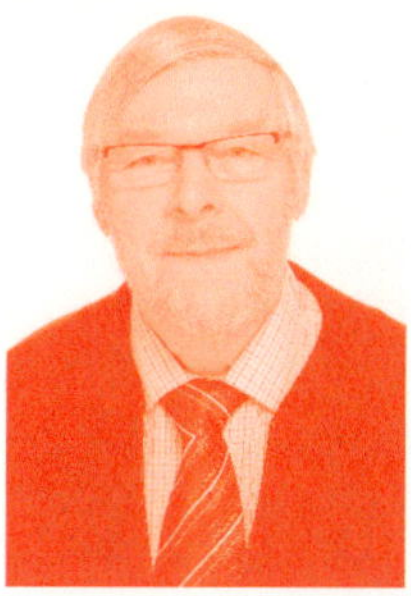
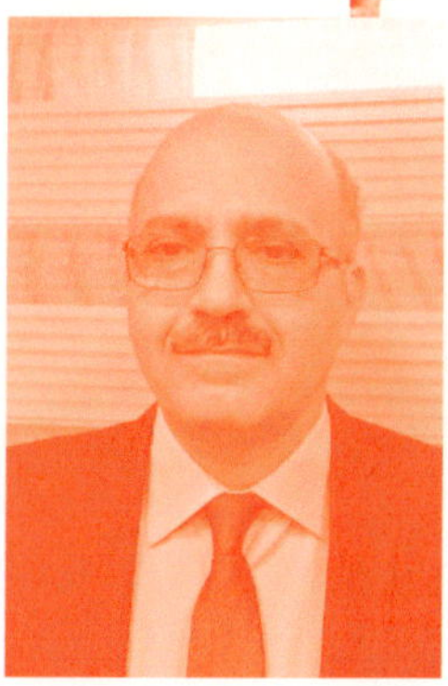
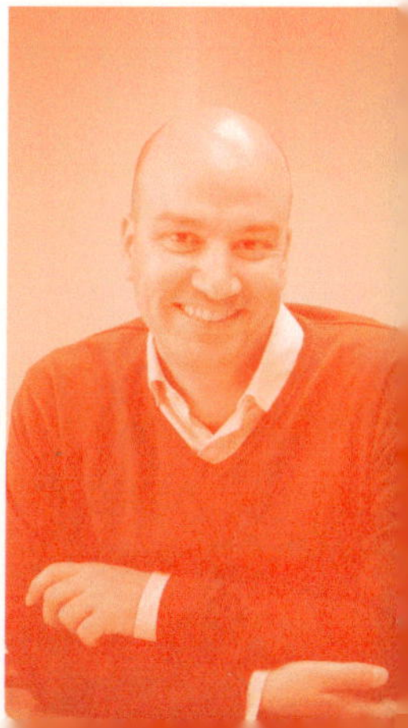
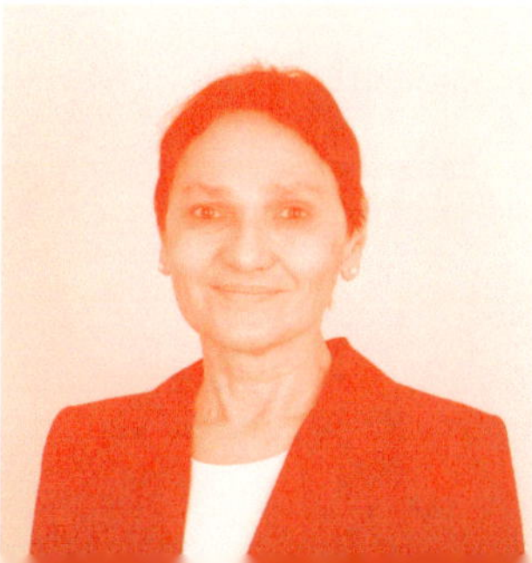

Esophagitis and Gastritis - Recent Updates
http://dx.doi.org/10.5772/intechopen.91500
Edited by Vincenzo Neri and Monjur Ahmed

Contributors
Adel. E. Ahmad Ganaw, Moad Ehfeda, Sohel Mohamed Jamal Ahmed, Arshad Husain Chanda, Zia Mahmood Awan, Qazi Zeeshan Ul Haq, Ali O Mohamed Bel Khair, Salem M Mustafa Jabira, Hossam Mohamed Algallie, Ahmed H. M. Almaqadma, Mahmud M A Ben Masoud, Edda Battaglia, Valentina Boano, Mario Grassini, Chiara M.C. Elia, Carlo Sguazzini, Maria Luisa Niola, Karam Salman Dawood, Israa Mamdooh, Daniella Kingsley-Godwin, Maria Jana Kingsley-Godwin, Joshua Godwin, Ljiljana Širić, Marinela Rosso, Aleksandar Včev, Vincenzo Neri, Nicola Tartaglia, Alberto Fersini, Pasquale Cianci, Antonio Ambrosi, Mario Pacilli, Giovanna Pavone, Monjur Ahmed, Mary Hägg, Thomas Franzén

First published in London, United Kingdom, 2021 by IntechOpen
IntechOpen is the global imprint of INTECHOPEN LIMITED, registered in England and Wales, registration number: 11086078, 5 Princes Gate Court, London, SW7 2QJ, United Kingdom
Printed in Croatia

British Library Cataloguing-in-Publication Data
A catalogue record for this book is available from the British Library

Additional hard and PDF copies can be obtained from orders@intechopen.com

Esophagitis and Gastritis - Recent Updates
Edited by Vincenzo Neri and Monjur Ahmed
p. cm.
Print ISBN 978-1-83969-059-4
Online ISBN 978-1-83969-060-0
eBook (PDF) ISBN 978-1-83969-061-7

Meet the editors

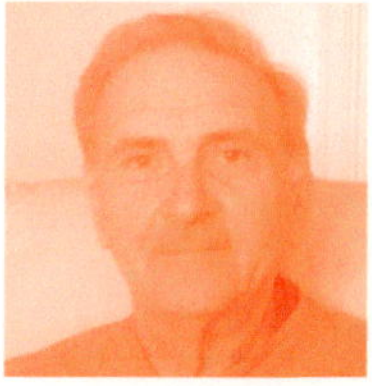

Vincenzo Neri is a former Professor of General Surgery (retired), Department of Medical and Surgical Sciences, University of Foggia, Italy. He also held positions such as Director of Division of General Surgery, Director of Residency School of General Surgery, Director of Department of Surgical Sciences, and President of Course of Degree of Medicine and Surgery at the same university. He also served as an assistant professor (1974–1982) and associate professor (1982–2001) at the School of Medicine and Surgery, University of Bari, Italy, where he obtained a degree in Medicine and Surgery and completed postgraduate training in General Surgery and Emergency Surgery. He obtained a diploma of "Maitrise Universitaire en Pedagogie des Sciences de la Santè" from the University Paris-Nord Bobigny in 1995. Dr. Neri's research interests include hepatobiliary pancreatic surgery, acute pancreatitis, and treatment of pancreatic and liver tumors. He has published research papers, reviews, congress proceedings, and book chapters. In the period 1991–2016, he attended the Hepatobiliarypancreatic Surgery Service of Beaujon Hospital, Universitè de Paris, Clichy. As part of the 2010–2011 ERASMUS Program, Dr. Neri developed a seminar on "Cystic Tumours of the Pancreas" at Ghent University, Belgium. He is a member of several scientific associations including Società Italiana di Chirurgia (SIC), International Hepato-Pancreato Biliary Association (IHPBA), European Association for the Study of the Liver (EASL), New European Surgical Academy (NESA), and Society of Laparoscopic and Robotic Surgeons (SLS).

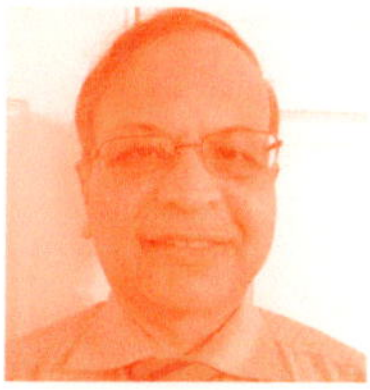

Monjur Ahmed, MD, FRCP, is an Associate Professor of Medicine at Thomas Jefferson University, Philadelphia, Pennsylvania, USA. He has been a practicing gastroenterologist for twenty-two years. He has a special interest in inflammatory bowel disease, eosinophilic esophagitis, gastrointestinal motility, and dysphagia. Dr. Ahmed also serves as an editor in chief for the *World Journal of Gastrointestinal Oncology*.

Contents

Preface

The functional role of the esophagus is motility, which is the motion that advances liquid and solid foods from the mouth to the stomach; there is no secretion activity. The term esophagitis refers to all inflammations and irritative effects on the esophageal mucosa. Common causes include acid gastric reflux, side effects of some medications, bacterial or viral infections, ingestion of strong acid or alkali solutions or solid substances, and so on. The clinical appearance of esophagitis can be characterized by heartburn, dysphagia, odynophagia, cough, nausea, vomiting, chest pain, or sore throat. In general, esophagitis, if untreated, can cause esophageal ulcers followed by scarring and narrowing or neoplastic degeneration. Acid reflux leads to gastroesophageal reflux disease, which is a complex clinical condition with some mucosal esophageal lesions with increasing severity (Barrett's esophagus). Usually, infectious esophagitis, by bacteria, viruses, fungi, or parasites, can occur in patients with weakened immune systems. Eosinophilic esophagitis is based on the excessive response to some allergens (milk, eggs, peanuts, etc.). The expression "gastritis" is the more discussed and ambiguous diagnostic definition of gastric clinicopathological conditions. In the current medical language, there is confusion regarding the definition of this pathology because the term "gastritis" is currently used indifferently for symptoms in the upper gastrointestinal (GI) tract or for endoscopic aspects and histological characteristics that can be referred to as gastric mucosal phlogosis, erosion, hemorrhagic lesions, or injury. We must remember that inflammation of the gastric mucosa should not present symptoms in the upper GI tract. Clinical and instrumental exams provide data that are difficult to correlate with each other. The symptoms that can be referred to as esophagogastroduodenal tract are epigastric pain, heartburn, and dyspepsia; endoscopy can identify various mucosal characteristics such as hypertrophy, friability, atrophy, and hemorrhagic and erosive lesions. It is important to underline the poor correlations between endoscopic mucosal abnormalities and histological features of the same lesions. In fact, for example, gastric mucosa described endoscopically as normal should show histologically severe signs of inflammation. On the contrary, evident endoscopic damage by drugs (e.g., aspirin) might turn out to be mild phlogistic lesions upon histological examination. We can conclude that the term gastritis should be used in the case of presence of phlogistic characteristics in the histological exam. However, the endoscopic examination has a fundamental role in the clinical scenario of gastritis because the microscopic evaluation is made on the mucosal biopsy. Endoscopic mucosal biopsies concern mucosal abnormalities such as erosion, ulcers, polyps, hemorrhagic lesions, endoluminal protuberances, or in cases of suspicion of *Helicobacter pylori* infection. Furthermore, the identification of *H. pylori* in gastric pathology has given a central role to gastritis. Gastritis includes acute and chronic inflammations of the gastric mucosa. The classifications of gastritis are based on histological data. Unfortunately, also within the histological field, it should be difficult to present a classification of gastritis because there are various criteria that can be followed. First, histological features of inflammation subdivide acute and chronic gastritis. Second, more detailed histological characteristics identify gastritis due to drugs, chemicals, infectious agents (viral, fungal, parasitic, bacterial), trauma, foreign bodies, tumors, autoimmune gastritis, vascular gastropathies, granulomatous gastritis, and so on. Finally, other histological features of the evolution and development of inflammation differentiate between chronic atrophic and hypertrophic gastritis (e.g., Sjogren's syndrome, Menetrier disease). In summary, gastritis is an inflammatory lesion of the gastric mucosa with various and numerous etiologic factors and histological features of inflammation; consequently, gastritis is a pathological state, but not a defined disease.

Peptic ulcers are based on acid peptic disorders, caused by the corrosive action of acid gastric juice on the vulnerable epithelium. This pathology can occur, through various clinical conditions, in the esophagus, stomach, and duodenum, or with ectopic gastric mucosa, in Meckel's diverticulum. Many peptic ulcers are due to the unregulated use of nonsteroidal anti-inflammatory drugs (NSAIDs) or infection with *H. pylori*. Additional factors include tobacco smoke and emotional stress, although the mechanisms are not clear. Ulcers may be defined as a pathological process of failure of the mucosal defense mechanism against the action of gastric acid and proteolytic enzymes, a secondary effect, in most cases, of NSAID drugs and *H. pylori* infection. Gastropathies are pathological conditions with the detriment of gastric mucosa without inflammation, which can be caused by an autoimmune reaction, drugs, infection, or chronic vascular congestive status, based on portal hypertension. Gastritis is inflammatory mucosal status due to damage from various agents such as drugs, autoimmune reactions, or infections. A particular kind of gastropathy is Menetrier disease, characterized by gastric mucosal hyperplasia, increased secretions, and loss of proteins. The clinical appearance of peptic ulcer disease is almost always abdominal pain. Epigastric pain, which may be diffuse or radiate to the back, is the characteristic symptom of the disease. Gastritis in most patients is asymptomatic. In Menetrier disease, in addition to epigastric pain, there is nausea, vomiting, loss of appetite, edema, weakness, and weight loss. The complications of peptic ulcer disease are hemorrhage, perforation, obstruction, and penetration. Hemorrhage occurs in 15% of cases and perforation occurs in 7% of cases. The penetrating ulcer erodes into the adjacent organs without perforation in the peritoneal cavity. Inflammation, edema, fibrosis, and scarring of the peptic ulcer cause outlet obstruction.

This book provides a comprehensive overview of esophagitis and gastritis and the many manifestations of these conditions. It begins with an introductory chapter that analyzes the complications of gastroduodenal ulcers. Section 2, "Esophagitis," discusses some topics of current clinical interest in the field of esophageal pathology. The first chapter in this section discusses the numerous infectious pathologies that can affect the esophagus. The second chapter in this section highlights the clinical characteristics of eosinophilic esophagitis. The third chapter examines extraesophageal manifestations and symptoms of esophageal disease. The section concludes with a chapter analyzing the innovative oral neuromuscular treatment of reflux caused by a hiatus hernia, as an aggravating factor in esophagitis.

The third section of the book, "Gastritis," includes several chapters on this wide and complex topic. The first chapter discusses the pathophysiology of *H. pylori*, as well as its infiltration through the surface epithelium and the body's induction of the immune response. The next chapter in this section discusses gastrointestinal pathophysiological testing for upper GI functional disorders. The last two chapters present two classic themes of gastroenterology: gastroduodenal lesions associated with portal hypertension and the anesthetic involvement in gastroscopy and colonoscopy.

Vincenzo Neri
Professor,
Department of Medical and Surgical Sciences,
University of Foggia,
Italy

Monjur Ahmed
Professor,
Department of Medicine,
Thomas Jefferson University Philadelphia,
Pennsylvania, USA

Section 1

Preamble

Chapter 1

Introductory Chapter: Complications of Gastroduodenal Ulcers

Vincenzo Neri and Monjur Ahmed

1. Introduction

In the past decades, after the widespread therapeutic use of antisecretive drugs (cimetidine, ranitidine, and proton pump inhibitors), the incidence of peptic ulcer disease showed a real and significant decrease. The treatment of the *Helicobacter pylori* infections contributed to these results, demonstrated by the reduced prevalence of these infections [1]. However, the expected reduction in ulcer disease complications did not clearly occur [2, 3]. It is possible to hypothesize a role in the widespread use, also as self-medication, of drugs with gastric injurious side effect such as acetylsalicylic acid (ASA) or nonsteroidal anti-inflammatory drugs (NSAIDs) and besides a role of inaccurate therapy for *H. pylori* infection [4]. Some research studies have shown the role of independent risk factors and a synergic action performed by the use of NSAIDs and the presence of *H. pylori* infection on the evolution of gastroduodenal mucosal impairment/ulceration, ulcer bleeding, and perforation [5]. There are also other significant risk factors of gastroduodenal ulcer occurrence and their complications, such as alcohol consumption, nicotine use, stress life conditions, immunosuppressor therapies, gastric acid hypersecretion states with hypergastrinemia, hyperhistaminemia, etc. [6–8]. In the gastroduodenal site, the mucosal transitional zones are the areas of major risk of development of peptic ulcer because of being exposed to damaging effects of pepsin, gastric acid secretion, bile, and pancreatic juice. The gastric ulcers are usually located along the lesser curvature, in continuousness with the fundus, site of the gastric acid production by the parietal cells. The duodenal ulcers habitually occur in the duodenal bulb and in the prepyloric area.

2. Pathophysiology of peptic ulcer and *H. pylori* infection

The pathophysiology of the gastric ulcers is characterized by the reduction of acid secretion, chronic gastritis, duodenogastric reflux of bile and pancreatic juice; on the other hand, in the duodenal ulcers there are elevation of gastric acid secretion, increase of parietal cell mass, and duodenal acid/pepsin charge. The identification of *H. pylori* infection as leading cause of peptic ulcer has completely changed the knowledge of the disease. Briefly we can believe that in the general population, the prevalence of the *H. pylori* infection as cause of peptic ulcer is very high, over 90% of patients with duodenal ulcer and 75% circa of patients with gastric ulcer. Furthermore, the *H. pylori* can be found in the gastroduodenal tract without disease. Usually the *H. pylori* is present in the patients with chronic gastritis

IntechOpen

that can develop in atrophic gastritis. The treatment therapies of *H. pylori* infection have been currently performed in the last decades and have shown effective, high recovery rate in peptic ulcer disease [9]. The usual way of the diagnosis is by endoscopic examination, and the medical therapy is currently effective. The complications of peptic ulcers, as bleeding, perforation, outflow obstruction usually require the endoscopic or radiological interventions or in some cases surgical procedures. The *H. pylori* causes damage, injury within the gastroduodenal mucosa followed by inflammatory response with mucosal ulceration. The *H. pylori*, in the gastric lumen, develops defense mechanism with production of urease enzyme, conversion of urea into ammonia and carbon dioxide, gastric acid tamponade, decreasing adverse gastric acidity. The alkalinization of the gastric setting causes decrease of somatostatine production, reduction of gastrin secretion, restriction. In summary, the disruption of secretory balance of gastrin is followed by parietal cell hyperplasia and rise of gastrinemia and gastric acidity [10]. The non-steroidal anti-inflammatory drugs (NSAIDs) and acetylsalicilic acid (ASA) accomplish peptic ulcers by local and systemic actions. These drugs, as acid, develop on gastroduodenal mucosal cells, cytotoxic action, and damage cell proliferation. The systemic action of NSAIDs develops by prevention of gastric prostaglandin output and its protective action versus mucosal damage of acydity by increase of mucus and bicarbonate production and increment of mucosal blood perfusion [11].

2.1 Briefly clinical appearance of uncomplicated peptic ulcer

Most evident symptom is the epigastric pain. This symptom can show a characteristic temporal cadency: the pain becomes worse in gastric ulcer after eating, but, on the contrary, it decreases over a period of time in duodenal ulcer after taking some meal. This traditional symptomatological distinction between gastric and duodenal ulcer is no longer the evident clinical data. Often the epigastric pain can be radiated to the back and linked to dyspepsia with the symptoms such as nausea, gastroduodenal reflux, heartburn, belching, etc. The diagnostic program for uncomplicated peptic ulcer encompasses gastroduodenal endoscopy as first step. In the gastric ulcer it is necessary to complete the examination with biopsy of the lesion for the risk of malignancy; endoscopy will be repeated, also with biopsy if it needs, to check for healing after the therapy. In the duodenal ulcer biopsies and further endoscopies are less required. In the diagnosed or suspected peptic ulcer, the test for *H. pylori* is routinely performed as mucosal biopsy for histological and microbiological control or with urease test [12].

3. Complications of peptic ulcer

The more frequent complication of peptic ulcer disease (PUD) is the bleeding (hemorrhage), followed by perforation and obstruction [13]. Some differences in the frequency among various complications can be found in the geographic distribution, due to amount of NSAIDs and ASA use, diffusion of *H. pylori* infection, lifestyles of the community. In fact the risk factors for complication occurrence in PUD, as hemorrhage or perforation, are the therapeutic use of NSAIDs or ASA, often as incorrect automedication, and untreated *H. pylori* infection.

3.1 Risk factors for peptic ulcer complications

In most cases peptic ulcer hemorrhage is connected with the use of NSAIDs and ASA. The risk degree is dose-dependent: the therapeutic employment of high dose is a greater risk factor for bleeding, compared with the use of medium or low dose of drugs [14]. The bleeding risk by NSAIDs is also drug-specific, for example, higher for Ketoralac and certainly higher for the synchronous use of aspirin and NSAIDs. Moreover these drugs play a real, concrete role in the occurrence of peptic ulcer perforation [15]. Likewise the presence of *H. pylori* infection is associated with the event of peptic ulcer complications as hemorrhage, but its role and mode of action are debatable in the development of the complication [16]. There are some hypotheses, sometimes conflicting, on the *H. pylori* actions: it was reported that the eradication of *H. pylori* infection reduces the bleeding complication; possible independent action or synergic interaction on peptic ulcer hemorrhage has been described; finally protective effect of *H. pylori* in the occurrence of hemorrhage was also communicated [17]. In some studies there is evidence of the absence of association between *H. pylori* infection and ulcer perforation [18]. Other risk factors for the development of the gastroduodenal ulcer complications, in particular bleeding, are the age over 60 years, associated use of corticosteroid and anticoagulants with NSAIDs, the presence of major comorbidities [19]. We could hypothesize a major incidence of peptic ulcer complications as bleeding or perforation in the patients with long history of ulcer disease without correct treatment, but there are not the studies comparing the incidence of complications before and after the wordwide introduction in the therapy of proton pump inhibitors and the eradication of *H. pylori* infection [16]. The pathological features of the peptic ulcer are an important factor that can modify the risk of complications: chronic ulcers, the penetrating character, and the great size of the lesions. The penetration into the gastroduodenal wall up to serosa, with sclerotic tissue, and erosive action on the blood vessels (sometimes of great size as gastroduodenal artery) are the pathological characteristics of bleeding and perforated peptic ulcers. All the complications of peptic ulcers require the preliminary therapeutic management: suspend ingestion of food, drinks, drugs; start the fluid resuscitation, immediate suspension, if previously foreseen in therapy, of ASA, NSAIDs, and also anticoagulant if possible, administer acid suppressive therapy with intravenous proton pump inhibitor (PPI), treatment of *H. pylori* infection, if certainly present [20]. The treatment of *H. pylori* infection actually decreases recurrent ulcers and the incidence of the complications. Consequently the therapeutic procedures for the eradication of the *H. pylori* infection (PPI, antibiotics per os, because the efficacy of antibiotics e.v. has not certainly demonstrated) have a fundamental role in the prevention of the complications and recurrences of the peptic ulcer disease [21].

3.2 Bleeding

The occurrence of hemorrhage complication is clearly higher than perforation. The evaluation of annual incidence of bleeding shows a large range of variation from 36 to 44%, followed by perforation with the range from 6 to 14% [22]. Bleeding complications can develop with various degrees of severity. Peptic ulcers cause almost half of all cases of upper gastrointestinal hemorrhage. The more serious events of bleeding usually are due to chronic duodenal ulcers; however, both gastric and duodenal ulcers have the overlappable trend to bleed. Gastroduodenal bleeding from peptic ulcer is a well-known clinical occurrence, in some cases with high morbidity. The reason of major severity of this complication in the duodenal ulcer is connected to anatomical condition: the ulcer situated on the posterior wall of duodenal bulb penetrates and exposes the gastroduodenal artery, which can be eroded followed usually by copious hemorrhage. In the other sites of the duodenal bulb, as anterior wall, there are no major blood vessels. The peptic ulcers in the second portion of duodenum, so-called postbulbar ulcers, are less usual than bulbar ulcers; however, bleeding complication is frequent also in this site. The clinical manifestation of bleeding is characterized by the amount and speed of hemorrhage. The massive and sudden bleeding appears with hematemesis, followed by melena, can cause hypovolemic condition and, in some cases, hypovolemic shock. Blood loss that develops less rapidly manifests with melena, also accompanied in some cases by hemodynamic alterations. In other cases continuous and moderate blood loss induces chronic anemia. Clinical data achieve the evaluation of the severity of hemorrhage and the general conditions, as hemodynamic stability, hypovolemic status, etc. The knowledge of these findings is central for the starting of urgent resuscitation therapy. However, the diagnosis must be completed by endoscopy to define the pathological features of bleeding ulcer, essential notion to perform the correct therapeutic approach: medical, endoscopic, surgical therapy. In the context of hemorrhagic complication, the control of possible active blood losses is necessary by checking stably the nasogastric tube, the stool, and the value of hematocrit and hemoglobin level. After the bleeding has stopped, rebleeding is possible, also within a short period of time. The urgent and current therapeutic approach in the patients with bleeding peptic ulcer includes fluid resuscitation, intravenous proton pump inhibitor (PPI) therapy, blood transfusions in some cases if necessary, therapeutic endoscopic procedures, if required. Usually this approach stops bleeding and cures the ulcer. However, the evolution of the bleeding complication is not favorable in the minority of patients, and the therapeutic resolution demands the surgical procedures. There are some clinical conditions that require surgery: patient with hypovolemic status and hemodynamic alteration not responding to powerful fluid resuscitation therapy; recurrent bleeding after early interruption, in most cases after unsuccessful further endoscopic treatment; finally in the patients with moderate, small, but continuous hemorrhage that needs prolonged fluid infusion and repeated blood transfusion.

3.3 Perforation

The global frequency of perforation in the evolution of peptic ulcer disease ranges between 2 and 10%. However, the sites of lesion, in the gastroduodenal tract, show different occurrence chance of the complication. The major frequency of perforation is in duodenal ulcer, reaching 60%; in the antral and gastric body site, the ulcer perforation develops by 20% [23, 24]. This clinical event is spontaneous. The free perforation in the peritoneal cavity causes upper abdominal pain; typically this pain is sudden, that is, the patient recalls precisely its onset and associates it with what he was doing. The first step of the peritoneal flogosis is a chemical peritonitis due to the gastric and biliopancreatic secretions. However, the reaction of peritoneal serous mitigates the gastroduodenal irritants with the light exudate, and the abdominal pain can ameliorate for a short frame time. This first phase is followed quickly by the return of the severe epigastric and then diffuse abdominal pain. The patient appears very suffering and reduces the movements of the abdominal wall with short breaths and bending off the thighs upward. The objective abdominal examination shows hypomobility of the wall, usually its board-like rigidity; with percussion tympanic sound instead of the normal dullness over the liver, because of the air leaking from the stomach; on auscultation, peristaltic sound is weak or absent. There are also atypical or less typical clinical presentations of peptic ulcer perforations. A small duodenal perforation with a small amount of gastroduodenal secretion flowing out along the right parietocolic douche can simulate acute appendicitis. Anyway in some patients the clinical appearance of perforation can be less pronounced with little symptomatological evidence and possible diagnostic pitfall. Finally, the so-called covered or sealed perforation is possible, due to the closure by the omentum or by the liver, or also the posterior, retroperitoneal perforation (epiploon retrocavity); these start with discrete clinical symptoms. However, the septic focus is active and usually develops in circumscribed peritonitis, as sub-hepatic or subdiaphragmatic abscess and also in generalized peritonitis [25, 26]. Within the laboratory findings, there is evidence of leukocytosis, with mild level in the early phases, after some hours more elevated. In the imaging studies, plain X-rays, with patient upright, of the lower chest and the abdomen reveal in most cases (plus than 80%) free subdiaphragmatic air. The clinical and this imaging data allow the diagnosis of ulcer perforation [27]. If the free intrabdominal air cannot be detected, the imaging study may be completed by US and CT. Both these exams can demonstrate also little amount of free air or fluid; the small fluid collection can be detected in the pelvic space. In particular there is evidence of the possible findings of little leaks through perforated ulcer by CT with oral contrast [27]. The early management of perforated peptic ulcer encloses fluid infusion, intravenous proton pump inhibitor, antibiotics with wide antimicrobial activity, and positioning of the nasogastric tube. The central therapeutic role in the peptic ulcer perforation is played by surgery, usually by mini-invasive approach, following one of several procedures of surgical ulcer closure [23, 24, 28]. The altered conditions in the patients with every free perforation are indication to urgent surgery. In the patients with little leaks through perforated ulcer or spontaneous closing of perforation, localized intraperitoneal inflammatory disease and well stable clinical conditions can be performed by nonoperative treatment by nasogastric tube, PPI, and antibiotics. However, the conservative management should allow a quick amelioration, that is, within 24 hours; but any delay in the improvement or also small deterioration of clinical condition requires urgent surgical procedure [29, 30].

3.4 Pyloric obstruction

The stenosis is the less frequent complication of the peptic ulcer, based on the evolution of the disease due to inflammation, edema, muscular spasm, followed by repair process with scaring. The detected frequency ranges between 5 and 8%. In detail, the development of this complication comprises various factors, some functional, other pathological. The functional factors are spasm, pyloric dysmotility, decrease of gastric motility, due to peptic ulcer disease; the pathological factors are inflammation, edema, fibrosis, and finally, scarring and stenosis. The first phase of dysfunction with edema and inflammation causes the reversible gastric obstruction, the following phase of fibrosis and scarring induces the irreversible obstruction [23]. The majority of patients who complain symptoms of gastric outlet obstruction have an history of peptic ulcer disease. The clinical appearance is characterized by anorexia, nausea, early satiety, epigastric pain, vomiting. This long untreated clinical condition is followed by weight loss and deterioration of general condition. A typical symptom is the decreased efficacy of antiacid drugs. This is the clue for the indication of altered acid gastric secretion condition: pyloric obstruction conducts to stasis with increase in the gastric pH, following rise of gastrin issue and overflow of acid secretion. Usually the diagnosis of stenosis and exclusion of malignancy are achieved by endoscopy, endobiopsy, and imaging exams, such as conventional radiography and CT scan. The initial medical management is based on re-establishment of hydroelectrolytic balance and gastric decompression by nasogastric tube for 48–72 hours. In some cases these procedures allow the resumption of oral diet and recovery of nutritional status. There are some studies that report the positive role of the treatment of *H. pylori* infection on the resolution of the outlet obstruction [31]. Also the NSAIDs use has been detected to cause gastropyloric obstruction and the favorable role of drug's suspension on the resolution of complication [32]. The operative treatment of gastric obstruction includes endoscopic procedures such as balloon dilation and surgical treatment as highly selective vagotomy with pyloroplasty, truncal vagotomy with gastrojejunostomy, or antrectomy.

4. Conclusions

Peptic ulcer complications are still remarkable medical problem. Although the current medical therapy of peptic ulcer, as PPI drugs, control of *H. pylori* infection, the decrease of the disease frequency was not followed by reduction of complications. Bleeding, perforation, and gastric-pyloric obstruction are evident. Proper treatment for bleeding encloses urgent medical approach and frequently therapeutic endoscopic procedures, usually followed by favorable evolution of complication. The failure of these therapies requires the surgery. For the perforation the central therapeutic role is usually played by surgical procedures; the opportunities for conservative therapy are limited. Gastric-pyloric obstruction can be treated with endoscopic approach and balloon dilation; in case of failure, the surgery is necessary.

Author details

Vincenzo Neri[1*] and Monjur Ahmed[2]

1 Department of Medical and Surgical Sciences, University of Foggia, Foggia, Italy

2 Department of Medicine, Thomas Jefferson University, Philadelphia, PA, USA

*Address all correspondence to: vincenzo.neri@unifg.it

References

[1] Wong SN, Sollano JD, Chan MM, et al. Changing trends in peptic ulcer prevalence in a tertiary care setting in the Philippines: A seven year study. Journal of Gastroenterology and Hepatology. 2005;**20**:628-632

[2] Sonnenberg A, Everhart JE. Health impact of peptic ulcer in the United States. The American Journal of Gastroenterology. 1997;**92**:614-620

[3] de Leest H, van Dieten H, van Tulder M, et al. Cost of treating bleeding and perforated peptic ulcers in the Netherlands. The Journal of Rheumatology. 2004;**31**:788-791

[4] Mc Carthy DM. Prevention and treatment of gastrointestinal symptoms and complication due to NSAIDs. Best Practice & Research. Clinical Gastroenterology. 2001;**15**:755-773

[5] Yuan Y, Padol IT, Hunt HR. Peptic ulcer disease today. Nature Clinical Practice. Gastroenterology & Hepatology. 2006;**3**:80-89

[6] Osefo N, Ito T, Jensen RT. Gastric acid hypersecretory states: Recent insights and advances. Current Gastroenterology Reports. 2009; **11**:433-441

[7] Phan J, Benhammou JN, Pisegna JR. Gastric hypersecretory states: Investigation and management. Current Treatment Options in Gastroenterology. 2015;**13**:386-397

[8] Peters MN, Richardson CT. Stressful life events, acid hypersecretion and ulcer disease. Gastroenterology. 1983;**84**:114-119

[9] Leodolter A, Kuling M, Brasch H, et al. A meta-analysis comparing eradication, healing and relapse rates in patients with *Helicobacter pylori*-associated gastric or duodenal ulcer. Alimentary Pharmacology & Therapeutics. 2001;**15**:1949-1958

[10] Mc Coll KE. Pathophysiology of duodenal ulcer disease. European Journal of Gastroenterology & Hepatology. 2012;**9**:S9-S12

[11] Musumba C, Jorgensen A, Sutton L, et al. The relative contribution of NSAIDs and *Helicobacter pylori* to the aetiology of endoscopically-diagnosed peptic ulcer disease: Observations from a tertiary referral hospital in the UK between 2005 and 2010. Alimentary Pharmacology & Therapeutics. 2012;**36**:48-56

[12] Mc Nully CA, Lehours P, Megrand F. Diagnosis of *Helicobacter pylori* infection. Helicobacter. 2011;**16**:10-18

[13] Wang YR, Richter JE, Dempsey DT. Trends and outcomes of hospitalizations for peptic ulcer disease in the United States 1993 to 2006. Annals of Surgery. 2010;**251**:51-58

[14] Lanas A, Garcia-Rodriguez LA, Arroyo MT, et al. Risk of upper gastrointestinal ulcer bleeding associated with selective cyclo-oxigenase-2 inhibitors, traditional non-aspirin, non-steroidal anti-inflammatory drugs, aspirin and combinations. Gut. 2006;**55**:1731-1738

[15] Collier DS, Pain JA. Non-steroidal anti-inflammatory drugs and peptic ulcer perforation. Gut. 1985;**26**:359-363

[16] Van Leerdam ME, Tytgat NJ. Review article: *Helicobacter pylori* infection in peptic ulcer haemorrhage. Alimentary Pharmacology & Therapeutics. 2002;**16**:66-78

[17] Lebenz J, Peitz U, Kohl H, et al. *Helicobacter pylori* increases the risk of peptic ulcer bleeding: A case control study. Italian Journal of

Gastroenterology and Hepatology. 1999; **31**:110-115

[18] Reinbach DH, Cruickshank G, Mc Coll KE. Acute perforated duodenal ulcer is not associated with *Helicobacter pylori* infection. Gut. 1993;**34**:1344-1347

[19] Skok P. The epidemiology of hemorrhage from the upper gastrointestinal tract in the mid-nineties—Has anything changed? Hepato-Gastroenterology. 1998; **45**(24):2228-2233

[20] Songur Y, Balkarli A, Acarturk G, et al. Comparison of infusion or low-dose proton pump inhibitor treatments in upper gastrointestinal system bleeding. European Journal of Internal Medicine. 2011;**22**:200-204

[21] Graham DY, Hepps KS, Ramirez FC, et al. Treatment of *Helicobacter pylori* reduces the rate of rebleeding in peptic ulcer disease. Scandinavian Journal of Gastroenterology. 1993;**28**:939-942

[22] Eisner F, Hermann D, Bajaeifer K, et al. Gastric ulcer complications after the introduction of proton pump inhibitors into clinical routine: 20 year experience. Visceral Medicine. 2017; **33**:221-226

[23] Behrman SW. Management of complicated peptic ulcer disease. Archives of Surgery. 2005;**140**:201-208

[24] Weledji EP. An overview of gastroduodenal perforation. Frontiers in Surgery. 2020;**7**:573901

[25] Moller MH, Adamsen S, Thomsen RW, et al. Preoperative prognostic factors for mortality in peptic ulcer perforation: A systematic review. Scandinavian Journal of Gastroenterology. 2010;**45**:785-805

[26] Zachary C. The Early Diagnosis of Acute Abdomen. London: Oxford University Press; 1972. pp. 79-84

[27] Grassi R, Romano S, Pinto A, et al. Gastroduodenal perforations: Conventional plain film, US and CT findings in 166 consecutive patients. European Journal of Radiology. 2004; **50**:30-36

[28] Kotha A, Kumar A, Kagalipura G. A study on surgical complications of peptic ulcer disease: A prospective study of tertiary care center. International Surgery Journal. 2020;**7**:408-413

[29] Soragne B, Jean F, Foulatier O, et al. Non operative treatment for perforated peptic ulcer: Results of prospective study. Annales de Chirurgie. 2004; **129**:578-583

[30] Donovan AJ, Berne TV, Donovan JA. Perforated duodenal ulcer: An alternative therapeutic plan. Archives of Surgery. 1998;**133**:1166-1171

[31] Gisbert JP, Pajares JM. Review article: *Helicobacter pylori* infection and gastric outlet obstruction. Prevalence of the infection and role of antimicrobial treatment. Alimentary Pharmacology & Therapeutics. 2002;**16**:1203-1208

[32] Boylan JJ, Gradzka ML. Long-term results of endoscopic balloon dilatation for gastric outlet obstruction. Digestive Diseases and Sciences. 1999;**44**:1883-1886

Section 2

Esophagitis

Chapter 2

Infectious Esophagitis

Daniella Kingsley-Godwin, Maria Jana Kingsley-Godwin and Joshua Godwin

Abstract

Esophagitis is the inflammation of the lining of the esophagus, which is characterized by its swelling and irritation. The esophagus is tubular structure which helps in the swallowing, and it links the back of the throat to the stomach. The swelling is commonly caused by acid reflux. Sometimes, this swelling can also be caused by infections. Infectious esophagitis can be set off by fungi, yeast, viruses, bacteria and other types of organisms. Anyone can get infectious esophagitis, but people with weakened or comprised immune system are more likely to develop the disease. Anyone can get it, but people are more likely to develop it if their immune system is weakened or compromised. The purpose of this chapter is to review the clinical manifestations, etiology, pathophysiology, histopathology, diagnosis, treatment/management, prevention, prognosis and other healthcare issues of infectious esophagitis.

Keywords: Infectious esophagitis, fungi, yeast, virus, bacteria, diagnosis, treatment, prevention

1. Introduction

Esophagitis is the swelling and irritation of the esophagus. Thus esophagitis refers to inflammation or injury to the esophageal mucosa. The esophagus is the tube that is used in swallowing and it connects the back of the throat to the stomach. There are many causes of esophagitis and essentially the presentation is similar which include retrosternal chest pain, heartburn, dysphagia or odynophagia [1, 2]. The most common cause of swelling and irritation of the esophagus is stomach acid that flows back into the esophagus, called gastroesophageal reflux, which can lead to erosive esophagitis. Other etiologies include radiation, infections, local injury caused by medications, pill esophagitis, and eosinophilic esophagitis (EoE) [3]. Patients with EoE may present with food impaction. If the esophagitis is severe and leads to strictures, fistulization, and perforation, patients may present with symptoms related to those entities.

In addition, infections can also cause swelling and irritation of the esophagus. Fungi, yeast, viruses, and bacteria can all set off the condition, called infectious esophagitis. Anyone can get it, but a person is more likely to develop it if their immune system is weakened [4].

The incidence of infectious esophagitis has become prevalent in immunocompromised patients with cancers and organ transplant because of their survival rates due to advances in medical practice and management techniques. The causative agent is normally *Candida albicans*. However, organisms like herpes simplex

IntechOpen

virus (HSV) and cytomegalovirus (CMV) have often been known to invade the esophagus. Patients with acquired immunodeficiency syndrome (AIDS) may develop more fulminant forms of fungal and viral esophagitis (including human immunodeficiency virus [HIV] esophagitis), accentuating the need for early diagnosis and treatment. The purpose of this chapter is to review the clinical manifestations, etiology, pathophysiology, histopathology, diagnosis, treatment/management, prevention, prognosis and other healthcare issues of infectious esophagitis.

2. Etiology

The causes of infectious esophagitis are many and they involve [5–13]J:

- Fungi, like *C. albicans*, which is the most common pathogen. However, other *Candida* group of organisms, for example C tropical, C galbarta and C parapsilosis have also been identified as rare causes of esophagitis.

- Other types of fungi such as Aspergillus, Histoplasma, Crytococcus,l Blastomyces etc.

- Viruses such as Herpex simplex (HSV), Cytomegalovirus (CMV), Varicella-zoster virus (VZV), Epstein–Barr virus (EBV), Human papillomavirus (HPV), Poliovirus etc. It is important to note that people infected with the human immunodeficiency virus (HIV), CMV, HSV, *Mycobacterium avium*-intracellulare are idiopathic in nature.

- Bacteria such as normal flora, *Mycobacterium tuberculosis*, Mavium-intracellulare, Saphylococcus, Streptococcus, Lactobacillus, Norcadia etc.

- Parasitic agents such as chagas disease, Trypanosama cruzi, Cryptosporidium, Pneumocystis, Leishmania donovani etc.

The risk factors of infectious esophagitis include antibiotics and steroids use, chemotherapy, radiation therapy, malignancies and immunodeficiency syndromes like the acquired immunodeficiency syndrome (AIDS). Additional diseases linked to increase in the incidence of Candida esophagitis include esophageal stasis, alcoholism, malnutrition, and advanced age. Occasionally, Candida esophagitis can occur in otherwise healthy individuals with no underlying esophageal or systemic disease [7–13].

Additional typical risk factors such as acute onset of symptoms such as dysphagia and odynophagia are also remarkable in some cases of infectious esophagitis. The disease may coexist with heartburn, retrosternal pain, nausea and sometimes vomiting. Occasionally, patients can present with abdominal pain, anorexia, weight loss and cough. Infectious esophagitis is frequently caused by *Candida* organisms. Other important causes include CMV and HSV infection.

Again, people presenting with generalized sepsis, low neutrophil counts, AIDS, burns, trauma etc., can have rare infectious esophagitis. Severe esophagitis with very deep ulcers and fistulous tracts to the mediastinum, pleural space, tracheobronchial tree, skin and other tissues can be due to actinomycosis. The appearance of characteristic sulfur granules on endoscopic biopsy specimens can confirm the diagnosis of infectious esophagitis. The most notable risk factor for infectious esophagitis in people with HIV is reoccurring low CD4 count. However, it has also been suggested that people can develop fungal esophagitis during the seroconversion phase of the process [5, 7–13].

3. Pathophysiology

Many agents like fungi, bacteria, parasites, viruses and other microorganisms can cause infectious esophagitis. The disease is more prevalent in immunocomprised people, but it can also occur in healthy people, including adults and children [13, 14]. The least common of all causative agents for infectious esophagitis is bacteria, but the most common cause of infectious esophagitis is .

The steps involved in the pathophysiology of infectious esophagitis include:

- colonization with mucosal adherence and proliferation is the first step in pathophysiology of infectious esophagitis.
- impairing the host defense mechanisms

Whilst *Candida Albicans* is a normal component of oral flora, it can also become a problem if their number increases, for example, with the use of antibiotics or if the patient is immunosuppressed because of treatment with corticosteroids. HSV is the most common cause of viral esophagitis, and it infects the squamous epithelium leading to vesicles and then ulcerations. CMV, Epstein–Barr (EBV) and varicella-zoster (VZV) are other viral causes of viral esophagitis.

Individuals may become susceptible to acquiring opportunistic infections like neutropenia, impaired chemotaxis and phagocytosis, impaired T-cell lymphocyte function and alteration in humoral immunity due to wide range of abnormalities in the host defense.

People suffering from various systemic diseases such as adrenal dysfunction, alcoholism, diabetes etc., and older citizens can be prone to catching infectious esophagitis due to altered immune function steroids, radiation, cytoxic agents and immune modulators can also lead to the impaired host immune function.

The mucosal protective barriers and antibiotics that suppress the normal bacterial flora disruption may contribute to the invasive ability of commensal organisms [14]. Categories of infectious are as follows [11–14]:

i. Fungal esophagitis, for example, Candida Esophagitis

ii. Viral esophagitis, for example, HPV esophagitis and CMV esophagitis etc.

iii. Bacterial esophagitis, for example, tuberculosis, actinomycosis etc.

iv. Tuberculous esophagitis as stated in point (iii) above

v. Other infections that can cause esophagitis

Fungal overgrowth in the esophagus, or impaired cell-mediated immunity or both can result in the development of *Candida* esophagitis.

The setting of esophageal stasis leads to cause of fungal overgrowth resulting from:

a. abnormal esophageal motility like achalasia

b. scleroderma or mechanical causes such as strictures.

Dysfunctional cell-mediated immunity can be caused by:

a. immunosuppressive treatment, for example with cytotoxic agents or steroids that might suppress both granulocytes and lymphocytes functions

b. Malignancy

c. AIDS

Candida esophagitis also associated with chronic mucocutaneous candidiasis, which is a congenital immunodeficiency state.

Diseases that interfere with esophageal peristalsis like achalasia, esophageal cancer and progressive systemic sclerosis may lead to fungal esophagitis.

Primarily, esophagitis caused by HPV is presented by small vesicle developments that rupture eventually forming superficial ulcers on the mucosa that are discrete in nature.

The host promotes healing of the ulcers in immunocompetent people. However in severely immusosuppressed people, the disease may progress from discrete areas of ulceration hemorrahgic esophagitis that is diffused. Candidiasis may heavily infect necrotic herpetic ulcers.

The esophagus is normally involved by erosion of concerned mediastinal lymph nodes abutting the esophagus in tuberculous esophagitis.

In addition, infection of the esophagus by bacteria occurs in the immunocompromised host, is usually polymicrobial, and derives from oral flora. This entity is underdiagnosed in severely granulocytopenic patients, given that bacteria are difficult to identify on routine histologic examination. In such patients, bacterial infection often coexists with viral or fungal organisms that are more readily detected. Suppression of gastric acid production (by proton pump inhibitors) may predispose to bacterial and fungal esophagitis. The diagnosis is made by endoscopic biopsy, and in these specimens, clusters of bacteria are mixed with necrotic epithelial cells. Treatment consists of broad-spectrum antimicrobial therapy.

Although infectious esophagitis is usually caused by fungal or viral organisms, other rare causes include Staphylococcus, Streptococcus, Klebsiella, Blastomyces, Cryptosporidium, *Torulopsis glabrata*, and *Lactobacillus acidophilus*.

4. Clinical presentation

4.1 Patient history

The history findings vary based on the type of esophagitis. Esophageal food impaction can be the initial presentation of proton pump inhibitor (PPI)-responsive eosinophilic esophagitis [15].

4.2 Symptoms

Immunosuppressed people are prone to developing infectious esophagitis. Fungi like Candida organisms and viruses such as HPV and CMV are the most common causes of infectious esophagitis. The diagnosis of infectious esophagitis is supported by immunocompromisation, steroid treatment, systemic disease or recent antibiotic use. Whilst some people may not have any symptoms of infectious esophagitis, notable symptoms of the disease are [1–15]:

- Experiencing pain when swallowing
- Having trouble swallowing
- Pain in the mouth
- Pain in the chest and heartburn
- Feeling nauseous or vomiting
- Feeling feverish or experiencing chills
- Loss of appetite, anorexia, loss of weights
- Coughing
- Pain in the abdomen
- Intermittent hematemesis

As the symptoms of infectious esophagitis may mimic other diseases, it is important that proper investigation and diagnosis are made in order to have better outcome for the patients.

In people with one or more predisposing factors for *Candida* esophagitis, it is often manifested clinically by dysphagia and/or odynophagia. Symptoms differ in characteristics and features that differ in intensity like mild/moderate achalasia to severe odynophagia, which makes it very hard for sufferers to eat food or swallowing. Some people may develop retrosternal pain or bleeding in the gut. However, some people do not have any symptoms.

Esophagitis caused by HPV is commonly present in immunosuppressed people with AIDS, existing cancer or long term serious diseases or people that had received steroids, chemotherapy or radiation treatments [13–15]. In healthy people with no existing medical conditions, herpes esophagitis can sometimes occur as acute self-limiting disease. Acute onset of severe odynophagia is usually present in people with herpes esophagitis. Difficulty in swallowing, pain in the chest and bleeding in the upper gut are other presenting symptoms in herpes esophagitis.

The development of severe odynophagia, dysphagia or both in people with AIDS is as a result of the manifestation of CMV. Evidence of CMV infection may be present in other organs and tissues like the colon, retina and liver in infected people. Patients may develop fear of eating sometimes in cases of severe odynophagia.

People with ulcers due to HIV normally show acute onset of severe odynophagia, dysphagia or both. A characteristic maculopapular rash may be visible on the upper half of the body if the ulcers manifest at the time of seroconversion.

People with advanced pulmonary or mediastinal tuberculosis or in immunodeficiency that have disseminated tuberculosis or other mycobacterial illnesses develop tuberculous esophagitis.

5. Diagnosis and differential diagnoses strategies

In considering the diagnosis and differential diagnosis of infectious esophagitis, it would be important to look at the diagnostic considerations and diagnosis considerations for the different types of infectious esophagitis in order to have understandings of the various issues to note for making decisions on the suitable treatments for better outcomes for the patients.

5.1 Diagnostic considerations

The possibility of a systemic illness causing the esophageal manifestations should always be considered (for example, AIDS, scleroderma, systemic lupus erythematosus (SLE) and pemphigus). Similarly, cardiac causes of chest discomfort should also be considered, and the appropriate treatment should be given. If the diagnosis is unclear, admission for further evaluation is suggested. Do not misdiagnose cardiac chest pain as esophageal pain. Pain can be similar, particularly in elderly patients and women.

Conditions that may mimic symptoms of esophagitis include the following [12–15]:

- Coronary artery disease
- Pericarditis
- Aortic aneurysm
- Nonulcer reflux disease
- Functional dyspepsia
- Stricture

5.2 Diagnosis considerations for the different types of infectious esophagitis

The diagnosis considerations for the various types of infectious esophagitis are discussed below.

5.2.1 Diagnosis of Candida esophagitis

Reflux esophagitis, herpes esophagitis, superficial spreading carcinoma and glycogenic acanthosis, may produce findings similar to those seen in *Candida* esophagitis. However, it is also important to note that elderly people who do have any symptoms of the esophagus and the more rounded appearance of the mucosal nodules of glycogenic acanthosis do indeed present with glycogenic acanthosis, but the candidiasis plaques are more linear in appearance.

A nodular mucosa of reflux esophagitis can also be present in patients. However, the nodules are difficult to identify than those found in candidiasis, and they are normally infectious with the gastroesophageal junction.

Multiple plaquelike lesions in the gullet are sometimes due to herpes esophagitis, which is normally linked to small superficial ulcers. Cancers that are spreading superficially may also present as a nodular mucosa with poorly defined nodular borders, leading to a confluent area of disease.

The plaques of candidiasis may resemble the insoluble effervescent particles and debris in the gullet. Hence the performance of a double-contrast study should be undertaken without the use of effervescent granules if infectious esophagitis is suspected.

5.2.2 Diagnostic factors for herpes simplex (HSV) esophagitis

Esophagitis due to the HSV can be identified by discrete superficial ulcers in the upper/mid gullet in the absence of the linked plaques, in the appropriate clinical environment. On the other hand, Candida esophagitis ulceration usually manifests on a background of extensive formation of plaque. Double-contrast investigations can be used in the diagnosis of Candida and herpes esophagitis without performing an endoscopy. It is also important to undertake endoscopic evaluation for confirmation of diagnosis when radiographic findings are ambiguous or when the problem do not respond to the treatment given to them.

Drug-induced esophagitis and Crohn disease are other causes of small superficial ulcers in the upper/mid esophagus, but these diseases can be differentiated from infectious esophagitis via detailed and careful patient history.

5.2.3 Diagnostic factors for CMV esophagitis

Endoscopy with biopsy is the most effective diagnostic tool for CMV. Large punched out lesions are seen in mid esophagus on inspection. Enlarged cells in the sub-epithelial layer with inclusions within the cells' nucleus and its cytoplasm can be seen in histological analysis of the lesions. Fluorescent staining with an immunoperoxidase stain is very specific in addition to the histological investigation. The diagnosis of CMV esophagitis cannot be made effectively with radiologic imaging tests like X-rays or CT scans alone, but they can be helpful in discovering of any resulting fistulae or strictures.

The presentation of large/giant ulcers in a patient may suggest the diagnosis of CMV esophagitis in AIDS patients because herpetic ulcers really becomes as big as those of infectious esophagitis, but giant/large ulcers can also be caused by HIV in HIV positive people.

Giant esophageal ulcers can also be caused by nasogastric intubation; endoscopic sclerotherapy; caustic injuries and oral medications, such as nonsteroidal anti-inflammatory drugs (NSAIDs), potassium chloride, and quinidine [13–15]. Efficient patient's clinical history is normally helpful in suggesting the correct diagnosis of CMV esophagitis [14, 15].

Again, CMV can be transmitted through many ways, which include mother to child transmission, which is common after birth and spreading of CMV through blood or sex, but transmission via tears, saliva, and skin contact is not common. Therefore patient education is very important in this regard.

5.2.4 Diagnostic factors for HIV esophagitis

It is important to rule out CMV esophagitis by performing endoscopy before confirming the HIV esophagitis diagnosis because most HIV ulcers are not distinguishable from CMV ulcers on the basis of just the clinical and radiological criteria alone. In addition, specimens from biopsy, brushings and viral cultures from the esophagus may be needed in order to be certain about the diagnosis and offer the patient the correct treatment.

During the period of transient chills, fever, malaise and rash of early infection with HIV, multiple, small, aphthoid lesions are observed on patients. In addition, giant deep ulcers measuring several centimeters can be seen later. Large ulcers may be complicated by fistula formation, perforation, hemorrhage, or superinfection in patients.

As most cases of HIV esophagitis responds well to oral steroids treatments, but CMV esophagitis is treated with toxic antiviral agents like ganciclovir, it is essential to differentiate between these infections. Hence endoscopic investigation should be undertaken before treating the patients.

5.2.5 Diagnostic factors for varicella-zoster virus (VZV) esophagitis

Severe esophagitis can be caused by Varicella-zoster virus (VZV), and finding its concurrent demographic lesions is extremely important to its diagnosis and also development of effective treatment plan for the patients.

On esophagogastroduodenoscopy (EGD), VZV has different features, which can range from infrequent vesicles of ulcerative lesions to a confluence of ulceration with necrosis. Epithelial cells with VZV display ballooning degeneration, edema and multinucleated giant cells with eosinophilic inclusion bodies on histologic investigation. In differentiating VZV from HSV, immunohistochemical staining utilizing monoclonal antibodies is usually helpful in the process.

5.2.6 Diagnostic factors for Epstein-Barr virus (EBV) esophagitis

Epstein–Barr virus (EBV) causes different syndromes in people. Crohn's disease and ulcerative colitis are common diseases that can be manifested by EBV, but the incidence and prevalence of EBV are still not well stated in both immunocompetent and immunodeficient people, hence, it should be seriously considered in any person presenting with symptoms of the esophagus. EBV esophagitis in an immuuno-competent individual is a rare occurrence, and thus represents either a primary infection, reactivation/reoccurrence, which si usually is characterized acute onset of symptoms and extensive ulcerative involvement of the upper/mid third of the esophagus. Oral hairy leukoplakia has similar histologic features of esophageal lesions linked to the EBV.

5.2.7 Diagnostic factors for human papillomavirus (HPV) esophagitis

Multiple epithelial lesions and cancers that are predominantly found on cutaneous mucosal surfaces are caused by the human papillomavirus (ahpv), which is a non-enveloped, double stranded, circular DNA virus. The virus has over 100 subtypes, and people with persistent HPV infection, especially those with many sexual partners are at very high risk for contracting more subtypes of HPV. At present, the HPV infection can be classified as non-genital/cutaneous; mucosal or anogenital and epidermodysplasia verruciformis (EV).

In some cases, the clinical lesions of HPV can be visibly identifiable, but in other cases, latent lesions of HPV may require testing for viral deoxyribonucleic acid (DNA) before confirming the diagnosis. In majority of the cases, HPV infections are latent and most lesions manifest as warts rather than malignancy in clinic.

Nowadays, the HPV has been identifies as the etiological agent for laryngeal, oral, lung and anogenital cancer. HPV subtypes six and 11 are low risk and usually manifest with the formation of condylomata and low grade precancerous lesions. However, HPV 16 and 18 are high risks that are responsible for high grade intraepithelial lesions, which progress to malignancies.

It is also crucial to note that HPV alone does not cause cancer, but it requires triggers such as folate deficiency, smoking, immunosuppression, and pregnancy and ultraviolet (UV) light exposure.

Esophagitis caused by HPV is an asymptomatic illness. Lesions of the disease are usually found in the middle to distal esophagus in patients and they may look like erythematous macules, white plaques, nodules, or exuberant frondlike lesions. The diagnosis of HPV esophagitis is made based on histology, and koilocytosis, giant cells, and cytologic atypia are visible on immunohistochemical stains.

5.2.8 Diagnostic factors for tuberculous esophagitis

The development of transverse or longitudinal sinus tracts or esophageal-airway fistulae can be as a result of the erosion of caseating nodes into the esophagus. People suffering from radiation esophagitis, Crohn's disease esophageal cancer or some sorts of trauma also display similar fistulae and tracts, but the clinical presentations of these patients normally portray the right diagnosis.

Intrinsic tuberculosis is very uncommon and it features of mucosal plaques, fistulae, strictures and ulcers. In a patient with tuberculosis, the development of difficulty in swallowing, cough and choking on swallowing indicates the involvement of the esophagus.

6. Treatment and management of infectious esophagitis

Treatment of infectious esophagitis is based on the patient's immune status, disease severity, and risk of complications [5, 16, 17]. The goal of medical care is to treat the underlying cause and minimize morbidity. The treatments strategies for the different types of infectious esophagitis are discussed below.

6.1 Treatment of fungal esophagitis

Antifungal drugs are normally used in the treatment of candidiasis in the throat, mouth or esophagus. The treatments for are categorized thus [18]:

- Active topical drugs such as oral amphotericin B, clotrimazole and nystatin

- Absorbable agents that are administered orally like fluconazole and itraconazole

- Agents like amphotericin B, flucytosine nad fluconazole that are administered parenterally

An antifungal medication that is applied to the inside of the mount between seven to 14 days is normally used in the treatment of mild to moderate infections of the throat or mouth. These drugs include clotrimazole, miconazole or nystatin. The most common treatment for severe fungal infections is fluconazole, which is an antifungal medicine that is taken by mouth or administered intravenously. If the patient does not respond to fluconazole, a different antifungal drug should be prescribed. The treatment for *Candida* esophagitis is fluconazole. However, another type of antifungal medication should be given to people who cannot tolerate fluconazole or who do not respond to the treatment with it.

It is important to note that treatment option chosen for a patient will depend on the severity of infection and the extent of the host defense impairment. For exam0ple, majority of immonocompetent people with fungal esophagitis can be treated with a topical antifungal medicine, which do not have adverse side effects, have only few or even any drug to drug interactions as the drugs are not absorbable in nature.

6.2 Treatment of HSV esophagitis

HSV esophagitis diagnosed at endoscopy can be treated with medications such as acyclovir (Zovirax); valacyclovir (Valtrex); famiciclovir (Valtrex), an acyclovir analog; and foscamet (for acyclovir-resistant cases). Pain relief medicines bought over the counter at pharmacies may also help in relieving pain caused be HPV esophagitis. Long term prescription of antiviral drugs can also be used in the prevention of the development of recurrent outbreaks of HSV esophagitis.

6.3 Treatment of CMV esophagitis

CMV is similar to HSV, as it is member of the *herpesviridae* family of viruses. Induction therapy for three to six weeks is used in the treatment of CMV esophagitis, but the optimal period of the treatment not yet well defined. The maintenance treatment for CMV is controversial. Overall, intravenously administered ganciclovir 5 mg/kg or foscarnet 90 mg/kg is the recommended treatment for induction therapy. As both ganciclovir and foscarnet are potent viral agents that have significant bone marrow and renal toxicities, extra care should be taken before they are prescribed to patients, by taking careful medical and drug histories form the patients, including any side effects they had had in the past.

It is also important to note that HIV esophagitis is treated differently from CMV esophagitis, but the two diseases cannot be simply separated on the basis of the clinical and radiographic results. Hence endoscopic investigation should be undertaken for a confirmatory diagnosis before patients are treatment in order to achieve a better clinical outcome. In addition, endoscopy has over 95% sensitivity in the diagnosis of CMV esophagitis.

6.4 Treatment of HIV esophagitis

HIV esophagitis is treated with oral corticosteroid therapy normally for over one month with antiretroviral therapy for HIV in contrast to CMV esophagitis.

6.5 Treatment of VZV esophagitis

Acyclovir, famciclovir or foscarnet (for acyclovir-resistant cases) are typically used in the treatment of VZV esophagitis.

6.6 Treatment of EBV esophagitis

Acyclovir is used in the treatment of EBV esophagitis. In order to suppress oral hairy leukoplaria, long term maintenance therapy may also be required for the patient.

6.7 Treatment of HPV esophagitis

No treatment is normally required, as HPV esophagitis is usually asymptomatic. Some medicines such as systemic interferon alfa, bleomycin and etoposide have been used in patients' treatments with variable outcomes.

6.8 Treatment of *M. tuberculosis* esophagitis

In the immunocompetent people, standard antituberculous therapy has been used in the treatment of mycobacterium tuberculosis esophagitis.

6.9 Treatment of bacterial esophagitis

In healthy individuals, infection by normal flora that is usually seen in immunosuppressed people are rare. Polymicrobial infections such as *Staphylococcus aureus, Staphylococcus epidermidis, Streptococcus viridans* and *Bacillus* species are often seen in patients with Bacterial esophagitis.

A broad-spectrum beta-lactam antibiotic with an aminoglycoside is used in the treatment of Bacterial esophagitis. It is also important to note that that the treatment is adjusted based on the results of response and culture.

7. Epidemiology of infectious esophagitis

The incident of esophagitis is low in children, but esophagitis is prevalent in adults [19, 20], and reflux esophagitis is the most common type.

The most type of infectious esophagitis is *Candida* esophagitis. Incidence of reflux esophagitis occur monthly in up to 44% of the general population, and up to 10% of people have daily symptoms of esophagitis [20].

In this section, we will look at the international statistics of the diseases and their prevalence in association with other disorders as described and discussed below.

7.1 International statistics

The prevalence of esophagitis is lower than the incidence of the symptoms of reflux sensation.

Patients presenting with symptoms of esophagitis to a General Practitioner (GP) in the United Kingdom (UK) show esophagitis rate in the range of 40–65%. The results of a retrospective review of results of over 800 diagnostic endoscopies in Hampshire, England, UK should that reflux esophagitis accounted for about 23% of all upper gastrointestinal diseases identified [21]. However, the incidence of infectious esophagitis is small in the studied population.

Another review of the Swedish National Register estimated that the prevalence of esophagitis diagnosed via endoscopy is about 5% or less in people aged 55 [22], and prevalence has also been estimated to be about 2% in other reports [23–25]. Again the incidents for infectious esophagitis low as indicated in the reports.

7.2 Prevalence in association with other disorders

In people with AIDS, leukemia and lynmphoma, the prevalence of symptomatic infectious esophagitis is high, but it is less than 5% in the general population, which is low.

As noted stated previously, the most common type of infectious esophagitis is Candida esophagitis. The second most common infectious esophagitis is HSV esophagitis, which has been reported in about 1% of immunosuppressed patients, and in as many as 43% of the patients in autopsy investigations [23–28].

Another etiological agent for esophagitis is CMV. A big percentage of the global population has been exposed to CMV and asymptomatic CMV infection is common around the world [29, 30].

CMV esophagitis was usually discovered on post-mortem analysis prior to the AIDS epidemic, and the first clinical case of CMV esophagitis was reported in 1985 [30].

CMV does not occur in immunocompetent people unlike HSV esophagitis, and the majority of the people with CMV esophagitis have AIDS [29, 30]. Since the advent of highly active antiretroviral therapy, the incidence of CMV esophagitis like those of other types of infectious esophagitis has declined among people with AIDS [29, 30]. On the other hand, there has been reported increase of CMV esophagitis in people who had undergone solid organ transplant, and in whom the onset of the disease was delayed due to the increasing routine of early CMV prophylaxis [31].

In AIDS patients in whom no other infectious etiological factors can be identified [32–36], giant esophageal ulcers have been observed [37], which have been called idiopathic HIV ulcers because they are believed to be caused by HIV, as electron microscopic investigation had confirmed the presence of HIV-like viral particles in the ulcer lesions [32–37].

Most patients have been found to have chronic AIDS with CD4 counts less than 100 cells/uL, despite the fact that some patients with HIV ulcers may have undergone recent seroconversion [38–41]. Ulcers associated with HIV have been under recognized generally, as it accounts for about 40% of all reported esophageal ulcers in AIDS patients [32–42].

8. Complications of infectious esophagitis

Unless a person has a medical condition that weakens his/her immunity, the complications of infectious esophagitis are rare, and they may include the following [43, 44]:

- Infection, which can spread to the other parts of the body
- Narrowing of the esophagus by scar tissue
- Bleeding from ulcers in the esophagus
- Perforation or fistula in the esophagus, including the formation of stricture
- Barrett esophagus, which occurs when the normal epithelium of the esophagus is replaced with columnar epithelium that is associated with cancer development.
- A serious and rare complication of perforation with mediastinitis
- Inability to swallow may cause volume depletion and weight loss
- If the gastric contents are refluxed up to the level of the larynx, laryngitis, aspiration bronchospasm and pneumonitis may occur.
- Failure to thrive and apnea may manifest in infants and children

9. Prognosis

The prognosis of infectious esophagitis is good with quick diagnosis, including effective and efficient treatment. Ultimately, prognosis depends on the underlying disease process.

Mild symptoms of esophagitis results in minimal morbidity and mortality. People with moderate-to- severe symptoms may suffer anxiety and lost time from work, which could lead to medical evaluations for more serious causes of pain.

Esophageal strictures (typically long, smooth, tapered areas of narrowing), malnutrition, and, rarely, perforation or bleeding can occur as a result of complicated esophagitis.

Barrett esophagus and adenocarcinoma are serious gastrointestinal complications of esophagitis in addition to strictures. In children, gastric content aspiration is a potentially serious respiratory complication that occurs frequently, that can be linked to apnea, pneumonitis and bronchospasm.

Odynophagia, malnutrition, dyspnea and pain may be as a result of severe esophagitis. On rare occasions, death may occur as a result of life threatening bleeding, but outcomes and survival in these patients are associated to the severity of their underlying systemic diseases.

Due to the fact that recurrence is a frequent problem in patients with reflux, many patients require maintenance therapy to prevent relapse of symptoms.

As *Candida* esophagitis is often self-limiting, many patients responds antifungal therapy [42, 43]. However, mycetoma, a fungus ball that causes obstruction may be formed from necrotic mucosal debris and fungal mycelia in the esophagus. The formation of strictures as a result of severe *Candida* esophagitis can also be seen in some patients. Rare fistula development into the tree of the bronchi, including ulceration and hemorrhage are other complications of infectious esophagitis, which will give poor outcome for the patients [43, 44].

Herpes esophagitis usually resolves spontaneously in immunocompetent patients within one to two weeks with conservative treatment involving analgesia and sedation. Rare complications of herpes esophagitis include perforation, tracheoesophageal fistulas, and dissemination to other organs.

Generally, most healthy individuals with infectious esophagitis recover within two to four weeks with proper therapy. However, recovery in people with comprised immunity (immunosuppressed people) recovery may take longer due to various factors.

10. Patient education and preventive measures

Clinicians should work closely with people who are recovering from infectious esophagitis and encourage them to keep all their follow-up medical appointments in order to monitor their progress and treatments outcomes.

The clinicians can suggest the following steps to patients that have ongoing symptoms of painful or difficulty in swallowing:

- Quit smoking and the use of tobacco and its products
- Stop alcohol and caffeine consumption
- Avoid over the counter drugs such as ibuprofen, aspirin and other non-steroidal anti-inflammatory drugs, which can irritate the esophagus
- Beverages and food that can cause heartburn should be avoided
- Try to lose weight if they are obsessed or overweight
- Eating smaller foods or meals more often
- Stop eating for three hours before going to bed

- Sleeping in flat position should be avoided, and the head of the bed should be elevated by several inches, i.e., six inch blocks. It is also important to discourage patients from sleeping with extra pillows as this may increase intra-abdominal pressure caused by people bending at the waist level.

The importance seeking early medical evaluation at the onset of symptoms should be emphasized to the patients and the general population in health education/health promotion campaigns. In addition, the importance of taking medicines with plenty of water while sitting upright in order to avoid the complications of drug-induced esophagitis should be highlighted to the patients.

Clinicians should also avoid the prescription of certain medications like alendronate in patients with obvious esophageal varices. It should also be noted that giving alendronate to patients who are cirrhotic could precipitate gastrointestinal bleeding from erosions over an esophageal varix.

11. Conclusion

Infectious esophagitis is a rare disease caused by viral, bacterial, or fungal agents or other organisms and infections. Patients who are immune suppressed, including people with granulocytopenia, lymphopenia etc., are usually prone to infections. Infection with *Candida* is the common cause of infectious esophagitis, but infections with HSP, bacteria and CMV are rare and accounts in up to 16% cases of infectious esophagitis in people with immunosuppression. Endoscopic observable ulcers with erythema, exudate and hemorrhage characterized bacterial esophagitis, and persistent symptoms include severe dysphagia and odynophagia, which may be a source of bacterial sepsis that will require prompt antibiotic treatment. Thus, infectious esophagitis causes morbidity in patients and careful diagnosis and treatment processes need to be followed in order to achieve better prognosis and outcomes for sufferers.

Conflict of interest

The authors declare no conflict of interest.

Author details

Daniella Kingsley-Godwin*, Maria Jana Kingsley-Godwin and Joshua Godwin
London Medical Academy, London, England, UK

*Address all correspondence to: daniellagodwin@ymail.com

References

[1] Mathieson R, and Dutta SK: [object Object]. Dig Dis Sci. 1983, 28: pp. 365-370, 1983.

[2] Baehr PH, and McDonald GB: Esophageal infections: Risk factors, presentation, diagnosis, and treatment. Gastroenterology 1994,106: pp. 509-532.

[3] Lewicki AM, and Moore JP: Esophageal moniliasis. AJR 1975; 125: pp. 218-245.

[4] Sheft DJ, and Shrago G: Esophageal moniliasis: Die spectrum of the disease. JAMA 1970; 213: pp. 1859-1862.

[5] O'Rourke A. Infective oesophagitis: epidemiology, cause, diagnosis and treatment options. Curr Opin Otolaryngol Head NeckSurg. Dec. 2015;23(6): 459-63.

[6] Quarto G, Sivero L, Somma P, et al. A case of infectious esophagitis caused by human papilloma virus. Minerva Gastroenterol Dietol. September 2008;54(3):317-21.

[7] Haron E, Vartivarian S, Anaissie E, Dekmezian R, Bodey GP. Primary *Candida* pneumonia. Experience at a large cancer center and review of the literature. Medicine (Baltimore) May, 1993; 72(3): 137- 42.

[8] Levine MS, Macones AJ Jr, Laufer *I*. *Candida* esophagitis: accuracy of radiographic diagnosis. Radiology March, 1985;581-7.

[9] Walsh TJ, Hamilton SR, Belitsos N. Esophageal candidiasis. Managing an increasingly prevalent infection. Postgrad Med. August, 1988;84(2): 193-6, 201-5.

[10] Kliemann DA, Pasqualotto AC, Falavigna M, Giaretta T, Severo LC. *Candida* esophagitis: species distribution and risk factors for infection. Rev Inst Med Trop Sao Paulo September, 2008;50(5):261-3.

[11] Vidal AP, Pannain VL, Bottino AM. [Esophagitis in patients with acquired human immunodeficiency syndrome: an histological and immunohistochemistry study]. Arq Gastroenterol October – December, 2007; 44(4):309-14.

[12] Bianchi Porro G, Parente F, Cemuschi M, The diagnosis of esophageal candidiasis in patients with acquired immune deficiency syndrome: is endoscopy always necessary?. Am J Gastroenterol February, 1989;84(2): 143-6.

[13] Sam JW, Levine MS, Rubesin SE, Laufer I. The "foamy" esophagus: a radiographic sign of *Candida* esophagitis. AJR Am J Roentgenol April, 2000;174(4):999-1002.

[14] Rothenberg ME. Biology and treatment of eosinophilic esophagitis. Gastroenterology, October, 2009; 137(4): 1238-49.

[15] Hiremath GS, Hameed F, Pacheco A, Olive A, Davis CM, Shulman RJ. Esophageal food impaction and eosinophilic esophagitis: a retrospective study, systematic review, and metaanalysis. DigDisSci. November, 2015; 60(11):3181-93.

[16] Dellon ES, Gibbs WB, Fritchie KJ, et al. Clinical, endoscopic, and histologic findings distinguish eosinophilic esophagitis from gastroesophageal reflux disease. Clin Gastroenterol Hepatol December. 2009; 7(12): 1305-13; quiz 1261.

[17] Jae Hyeuk Choi, Chang Geun Lee, Yun Jeong Lim et al. "Prevalence and Risk Factors of Esophageal Candidiasis in Healthy Individuals: A Single Center Experience in Korea" Published at:

https://www.researchgate.net/figure/Esophageal-candidiasis-A-Endoscopic-finding-multiple- whitish-plaques-were-identified figl 233888417. Accessed: 2021 – 04 - 07.

[18] Wilheim AB, Miranda-Filho Dde B, Nogueira RA, Rego RS, Lima Kde M, Pereira LM. The resistance to fluconazole in patients with esophageal candidiasis. Arq Gastroenterol 2009; (1):32-37.

[19] Prasad GA, Alexander J A, Schleck CD, et al. Epidemiology of eosinophilic esophagitis over three decades in Olmsted County, Minnesota. CLin Gastroenterol Hepatol October, 2009; 7(10): 1055-61.

[20] Nurko S, Rosen R, Furuta GT Esophageal dysmotility in children with eosinophilic esophagitis: a study using prolonged esophageal manometry. Am J Gastroenterol December. 2009; 104(12):3050-7.

[21] McColl KE Review article: *Helicobacter pylori* and gastro-oesophageal reflux disease-the European perspective. Aliment Pharmacol Ther. , December, 2004; 20 Suppl 8:36-9.

[22] The Swedish National Patient Register. https://www.lupop.lu.se/lupop-researchers/population-data-outside-lund-university/swedish-registers/swedish-national-patient-register . Accessed: 2021 – 04 - 07.

[23] Chen LI, Chang JM, Kuo MC, Hwang SJ, Chen HC. Combined herpes viral and *Candida*l esophagitis in a CAPD patient: case report and review of literature. Am J Med Sci. March, 2007; 333(3): 191-3.

[24] DeGaeta L, Levine MS, Guglielmi GE, Raffensperger EC, Laufer I. Herpes esophagitis in an otherwise healthy patient AJR Am J Roentgenol January, 1985; 144(6): 1205-6.

[25] Levine MS, Laufer 1, Kressel HY, Friedman HM. Herpes esophagitis. AJR Am J Roentgenol May, 1981; 136(5): 863-6.

[26] Levine MS, Loevner LA, Saul SH, Rubesin SE, Herlinger H, Laufer I. Herpes esophagitis: sensitivity of double-contrast esophagography. AJR Am J Roentgenol July, 1988; 151(1): 57-62.

[27] Shortsleeve MJ, Levine MS. Herpes esophagitis in otherwise healthy patients: clinical and radiographic findings. Radiology March, 1992; 182(3): 859-61.

[28] Borowitz SM Diagnosis: herpes simplex esophagitis. Clin Pediatr (Phila) July, 2007; 46(6):557-9.

[29] Geagea A, Cellier C. Scope of drug-induced, infectious and allergic esophageal injury. Cttrr Opin Gastroenterol July, 2008; 24(4) 496-501.

[30] Baroco AL, Oldfield EC. Gastrointestinal cytomegalovirus disease in the immunocompromised patient. Curr Gastroenterol Rep. August, 2008; 10(4):409-16.

[31] Buckner FS, Pomeroy C. Cytomegalovirus disease of the gastrointestinal tract in patients without AIDS Clin Infect Dis. October, 1993; 17(4):644-56.

[32] Vidal AP, Pannain VL, Bottino AM. [Esophagitis in patients with acquired human immunodeficiency syndrome: an histological and immunohistochemistry study], Arq Gastroenterol October - December. 2007; 44(4):309-14.

[33] Bonacini M, Young T, Laine L. Histopathology of human immunodeficiency virus-associated

esophageal disease. Am J Gastroenterol April, 1993; 88(4):549-51.

[34] Bonacini M, Young T, Laine L. The causes of esophageal symptoms in human immunodeficiency virus infection. A prospective study of 110 patients. Arch Intern Med. August, 1991; 151(8): 1567-72.

[35] Calore EE, Cavaliere JM, Perez NM, Campos Sales PS, Wamke KO. Esophageal ulcers in AIDS. Pathologica 89(2):155-8.

[36] Edwards P, Wodak A, Cooper DA, Thompson IL, Penny R The gastrointestinal manifestations of AIDS. AustNZJMed. April, 1997; 20(2). 141-8, April, 1990.

[37] Levine MS, Loercher G, Katzka DA, Herlinger H, Rubesin SE, Laufer I. Giant, human immunodeficiency virus-related ulcers in the esophagus. Radiology August. 1991; 180(2):323-6.

[38] Levine MS, Woldenberg R, Herlinger H, Laufer I. Opportunistic esophagitis in AIDS: radiographic diagnosis. Radiology! December, 1987; 65(3). 815-20.

[39] Raufman JP. Infectious esophagitis in AIDS: what have we learned in the last decade?. Am J Gastroenterol November, 1995; 90(11): 1914-5.

[40] Sor S, Levine MS, Kowalski TE, Laufer I, Rubesin SE, Herlinger H. Giant ulcers of the esophagus in patients with human immunodeficiency virus: clinical, radiographic, and pathologic findings. Radiology February, 1995; 194(2):447-51.

[41] Villanueva JL, Torre-Cisneros J, Jurado R, et al. Leishmania esophagitis in an AIDS patient: an unusual form of visceral leishmaniasis. Am J Gastroenterol February, 1994; 89(2):273-5.

[42] Yangco BG, Kenyon VS. Epidemiology and infectious complications of human immunodeficiency virus antibody positive patients. AdvExpMedBiol. 1993; 335:235-40.

[43] Howden CW, Homung C A. A systematic review of the association between Barrett's esophagus and colon neoplasms. Am J Gastroenterol October, 1995; 90(10):1814-9.

[44] Mimidis K, Papadopoulos V, Margaritis V, et al. Predisposing factors and clinical symptoms in HIV-negative patients with *Candida* oesophagitis: are they always present?. IntJ Clin Pract February, 2005; 59(2):210-3.

Chapter 3

Eosinophilic Esophagitis in 2021

Monjur Ahmed

Abstract

Eosinophilic esophagitis also known as asthma of the esophagus is a food-related allergic disorder of the esophagus widely distributed all over the world. The incidence and prevalence of eosinophilic esophagitis have been increasing over the last few decades. The pathogenesis of this entity is now better understood and three distinct endotypes have been defined for better management strategy. Diagnosis is made on the basis of clinical symptoms followed by endoscopy with biopsy. Drugs, diet and endoscopic dilation are the current modalities of treatment. IL-4 and IL-13 inhibitors have been found to be promising in clinical trials.

Keywords: eosinophilic esophagitis, asthma of esophagus, dysphagia, food bolus impaction, esophageal eosinophilia, esophageal stricture

1. Introduction

Eosinophilic esophagitis (EoE) is a chronic immune/allergy mediated disease of the esophagus characterized by esophageal eosinophilia (presence of ≥15 eosinophils/high power field in at least 1 esophageal biopsy.), esophageal dysfunction (dysphagia, food impaction) and characteristic endoscopic features [1]. To establish the diagnosis, other causes of esophageal eosinophilia must be excluded. In 1989, EoE was first recognized as a distinct clinical entity by Attwood et al. [2]. Now there is an epidemic of EoE in the western world. EoE is increasingly being recognized and diagnosed in our clinical practice both in the acute and chronic settings. EoE has distinct clinical epitopes, diagnostic and treatment protocol. The epidemiology, pathogenesis, pathology, clinical feature, investigations, management and prognosis will be described in this chapter.

2. Epidemiology

The disease is more common in Caucasian population with a male to female ratio of 3:1 [3]. Eosinophilic esophagitis has also been seen in African Americans, Asians and Hispanic population. The disease is increasingly being recognized over the last few decades. The current incidence is 5 to 10 cases per 100,000 population, and the current prevalence is 0.5 to 1 case per 1000 population in North America, Europe and Australia [4]. The disease can affect both children and adults. In adults, EoE is more commonly seen in males than in females and the average age of patients with EoE is between 30 and 50 years. Most of the patients with EoE have personal history of allergic disorders like bronchial asthma, allergic rhinitis, allergic conjunctivitis or food allergy.

3. Pathogenesis

Exposure of the esophagus to food and aeroallergens in genetically predisposed individuals may initiate the process of eosinophilic esophagitis although the exact mechanism is currently unknown [5]. Foods most commonly implicated in EoE are: Milk, egg, wheat, soy, peanuts, beans, rye and beef. Genomewide association analysis (GWAS) suggested that CAPN14 at 2p23 locus is upregulated after epithelial exposure to interleukin (IL)13 [6]. Recently, epithelialderived cytokine thymic stromal lymphopoietin (*TSLP*) gene at 5q22 locus has been identified as a candidate gene in

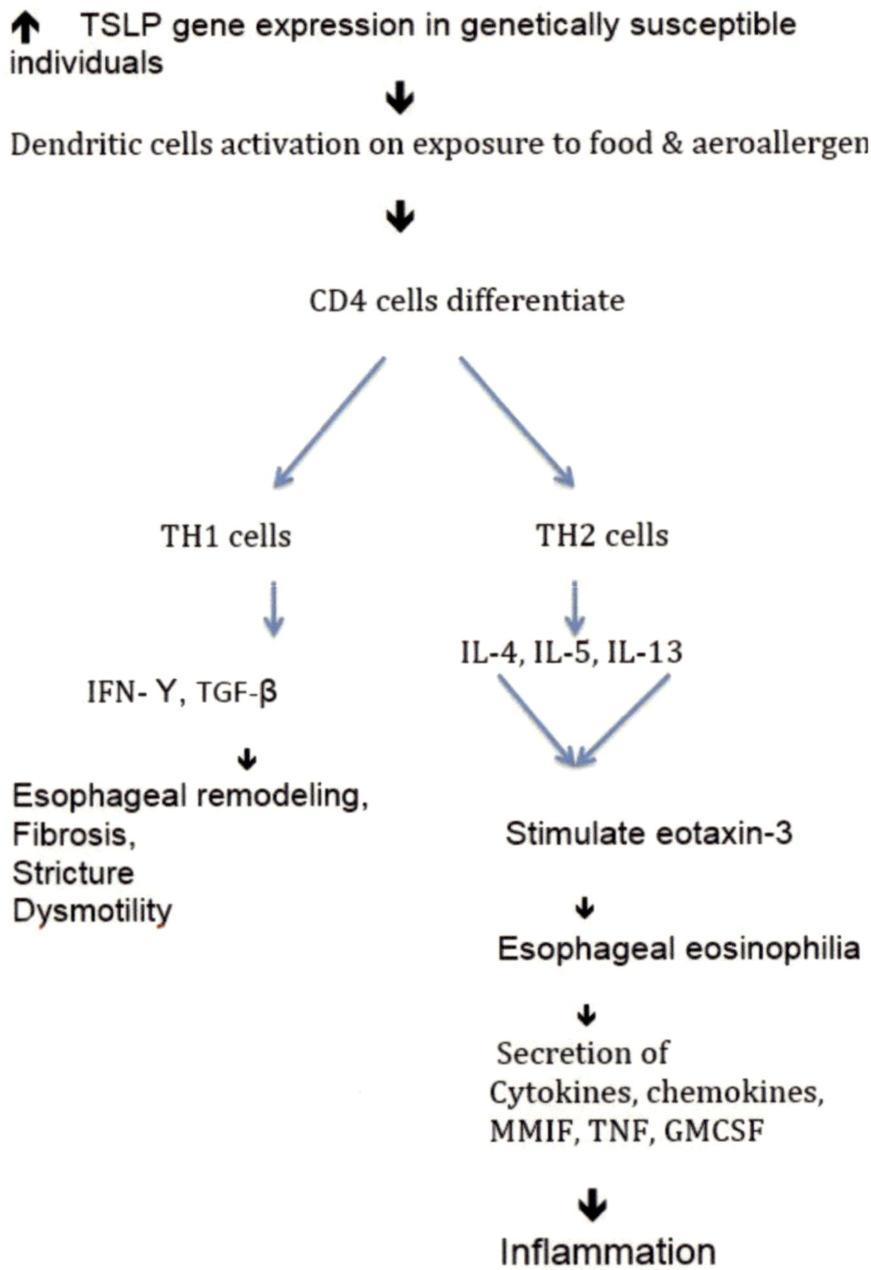

Figure 1.
Pathogenesis of EoE.

a multicenter GWAS. There is an increased expression of TSLP in patients with EoE. TSLP activates dendritic cells (antigen presenting cells). Food allergen is initially recognized by antigen presenting cells which differentiate CD4 cells into TH1 cells and TH2 cells. TH1 cells secrete interferonγ (IFN-ϒ) and transforming growth factorβ (TGF-β). TH2 cells secrete IL4, IL5 and IL13. There is also single nucleotide polymorphism (SNP) in this TSLP receptor gene in male patients with EoE. This gene is found on the pseudoautosomal region on Xp22.3 and Yp11.3. This finding may explain increased prevalence of EoE in male patients. There is also a suggestion of second hit for the development of EoE. Tolllike receptor3 (TLR3) can recognize double-stranded RNA (found in some viruses) and can induce TSLP [7]. IL5 is responsible for eosinophilic infiltration, growth and survival. Eosinophils secrete various inflammatory cytokines and chemokines including macrophage migration inhibitory factor (MMIF), tumor necrosis factor (TNF), granulocytemonocyte colony stimulating factors (GMCSF) and toxic granules [8]. TGF-β1 is a profibrotic molecule and helps in remodeling of the esophagus in EoE. This may lead to esophageal luminal narrowing, stricture formation and dysmotility. Eotaxin3 is a strong chemotactic agent for esophageal eosinophilia. A single nucleotide polymorphism in the human *eotaxin-3* gene was associated with disease susceptibility. IL4 and IL13 secreted by TH2 can stimulate eotaxin3. In telomeraseimmortalized esophageal squamous cells of EoE patients, IL4 stimulated eotaxin3 secretion was blocked by PPI omeprazole and lansoprazole [9]. This may explain PPI responsiveness of esophageal eosinophilia. Twin and family studies suggest that there is not only increased prevalence of EoE in male sex but also in monozygotic twins and other family member [10]. The pathogenesis of EoE is shown in a flow diagram in **Figure 1**.

4. Pathology

The major features (**Figure 2**) include infiltration of numerous eosinophils (usually >15 per high power field) into the squamous epithelium, layering of eosinophils on the surface layer and eosinophilic microabscess formation (clusters of ≥4 eosinophils). Often necrotic squamous cells are also seen on the surface layer [11]. Minor features include chronic inflammatory infiltrate into the lamina propria with fibrosis of the lamina propria [12], hyperplasia of muscular layers and basal epithelial cells with lengthening of lamina propria papillae, and intercellular edema. One study showed plenty of IgG4containing plasma cells in the lamina propria [13]. The pathological changes are patchy in distribution, and generally affect the whole

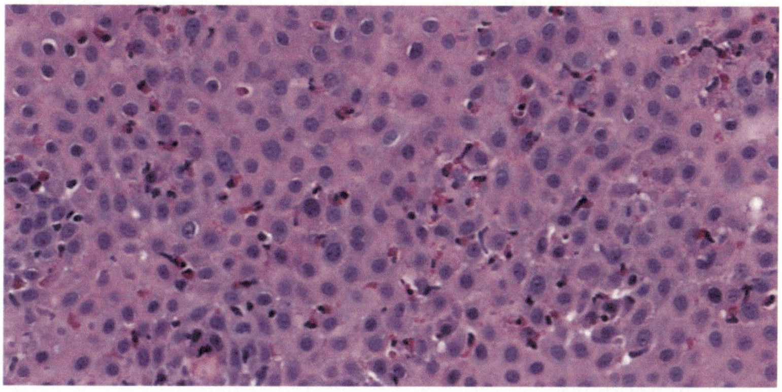

Figure 2.
HE staining showing esophageal eosinophilia.

length of the esophagus. None of the histologic findings is specific for eosinophilic esophagitis. Esophageal eosinophilia can be found in a variety of disorders including gastroesophageal reflux disease (GERD), eosinophilic gastroenteritis, hypereosinophilic syndrome, Crohn's disease, connective tissue diseases, drug hypersensitivity, parasitic and fungal infections and achalasia. In clinical practice, the real challenge comes to differentiate EoE from GERD [14]. Eosinophilic degranulation is seen more profoundly in EoE than in GERD biopsy specimen [15]. In EoE, the eosinophilic inflammation extends beyond mucosa into the submucosa and muscularis propria.

5. Clinical feature

Patients with eosinophilic esophagitis generally present with solid food dysphagia or esophageal food impaction requiring endoscopic removal of food bolus as an emergency case [16]. In one study, EoE was found in 9% of all cases of esophageal food impaction [17]. Commonly, the diagnosis is suspected after a first episode of esophageal food impaction and biopsy showing esophageal eosinophilia. Less commonly, patients present with heartburn and chest pain mimicking gastroesophageal reflux disease. One study found that gender was an important factor in the initial clinical presentation of eosinophilic esophagitis. Men presented with dysphagia and esophageal food impaction more commonly than women. Women presented with heartburn and chest pain more commonly than men [18]. Diffuse narrowing of the esophageal lumen has been seen in clinical practice as a result of chronic inflammation and fibrosis. Esophageal mucosa is friable in EoE, and as a result, esophageal mucosal tear and esophageal perforation can occur during endoscopic esophageal foreign body removal and during esophageal stricture dilation [19]. As aeroallergens play an important role in the pathogenesis, EoE is diagnosed more frequently when the environmental pollen counts (grass, trees and weeds) are high; the highest percentage of EoE occurs in the Spring and the lowest percentage in the Winter [20]. The diagnosis of EoE is not increased in the summer months [21].

6. Diagnostic tests

6.1 Laboratory (lab) tests

There is no single Lab test that can support the diagnosis of EoE. Mild peripheral eosinophilia may or may not be present. Peripheral eosinophilia, elevated serum eosinophilderived neurotoxin and eotaxin3 (CCL26) may have the potential to act as a biomarker for monitoring EoE [22].

6.2 Endoscopy

The esophageal mucosa may look normal in 7–10% of cases of EoE [23]. A variety of nonspecific features of inflammation can be seen in EoE during endoscopy. The five major endoscopic features of EoE as per EoE endoscopic reference score (EREFS) are edema, rings (**Figure 3**), exudates, furrows and strictures [24]. Edema is identified by loss of vascular markings and mucosal pallor. Transient concentric rings or trachealization may indicate esophageal longitudinal muscle contraction [25] and fixed rings may indicate fibrous stricture formation due to tissue remodeling. Exudates or white spots or white plaques may mimic candida esophagitis, histologically they are eosinophilic microabscesses. Furrows are vertical lines running parallel to the axis of the esophagus probably due to epithelial edema.

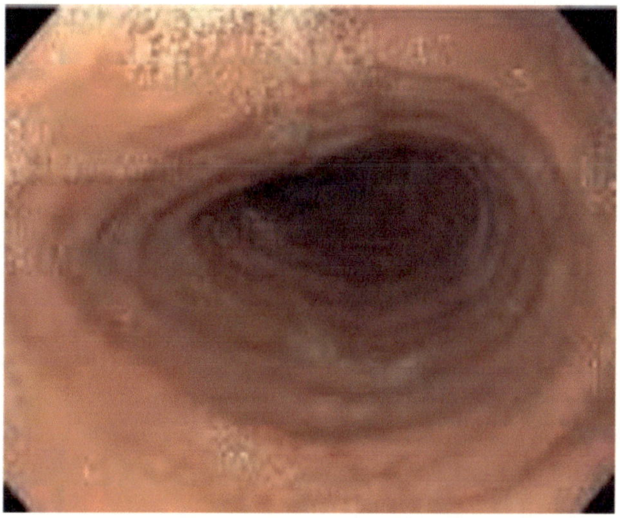

Figure 3.
Endoscopy showing multiple esophageal rings.

Chronic eosinophilic esophagitis may lead to long segment or short segment stricture. Narrowcaliber esophagus due to luminal narrowing of most of the esophagus is infrequently seen in EoE. Crepe paper esophagus occurs due to esophageal mucosal fragility and is recognized by a mucosal tear that occurs during passage of a diagnostic endoscope but neither during endoscope withdrawal nor after esophageal dilation. Although more than one of the above endoscopic findings can be seen in the same patient, none of them is specific for EoE. Recently, esophageal "pull" sign (substantial resistance and mucosal tenting during pulling of the biopsy forcep) was found to be highly specific and responsive to successful therapy in EoE patients [26].

Current recommendation is to take at least 2 to 4 biopsies from both proximal and distal halves of the esophagus (5 cm above GE junction) and also to take targeted biopsies from abnormal mucosa, *i.e.,* exudates, rings, edema, furrows and strictures. Gastric and duodenal biopsies should also be taken to evaluate eosinophilic gastroenteritis.

7. Barium swallow

Imaging studies are generally not done to diagnose EoE. Barium swallow may show normal esophagus. Sometimes featureless narrowcaliber esophagus, ringed esophagus, and isolated esophageal stricture are seen in EoE. But none is pathognomonic of EoE.

8. Esophageal manometry

Generally normal peristalsis is seen in EoE. Prolonged esophageal manometry and pHmetry showed ineffective esophageal peristalsis in children with EoE [27]. Twenty-four hours pH study would be normal in EoE unless there is coexistent GERD.

9. Echoendoscopy

Echoendoscopy may show hypoechogenesity and thickening of all the layers of the esophageal wall due to inflammation and edema [28].

10. Endotyping

In 2018, Consortium of Eosinophilic Gastrointestinal Disease Researchers analyzed endoscopic and histological features in patients with EoE using eosinophilic esophagitis diagnostic panel (EDP) which is a set of 96 informative transcripts. The EoE endoscopic reference score (EREFS), EoE histology scoring system (HSS), quantification of esophageal eosinophils and molecular features were assessed. The EDP identified clear signature of 3 distinct endotypes of EoE [29]:

1. Endotype 1 (EoEe1): It is the mild endotype. It is associated with relatively mild endoscopic (almost normal appearing esophagus), histologic and molecular changes. It is inversely associated with history of esophageal dilation. It represents 35% of all EoE patients.

2. Endotype 2 (EoEe2): It is the Inflammatory and steroid-refractory endotype. It is associated with esophagitis due to the highest expression of inflammatory cytokines. It has also the highest expression of steroid responding genes. It represents 29% of all EoE patients.

3. Endotype 3: It is the fibrostenotic and adult onset endotype. It is associated with narrow-caliber esophagus. It has the highest degree of endoscopic and histological severity and the lowest expression of epithelial differentiation genes. It represents 36% of all EoE patients.

10.1 Diagnostic criteria of EoE

1. Symptoms of esophageal dysfunction such as dysphagia, food impaction.

2. Characteristic endoscopic features: edema, rings, exudates, furrows and strictures (EREFS).

3. Esophageal eosinophilia i.e. > 15 eosinophils per high power field.

4. Exclusion of other causes of esophageal eosinophilia.

11. Management

Firm diagnosis of EoE is essential before offering any treatment. Symptomatic esophageal eosinophilia is now considered as EoE when other secondary/non-EoE causes are excluded [30]. Few years ago, the term proton pump inhibitor responsive esophageal eosinophilia (PPI REE) was used [31] but EoE and PPIREE are indistinguishable clinically, endoscopically and pathologically. The term PPI-REE is no longer used at the present time. The main aim of treatment of EoE is not only clinical improvement but also histological improvement to prevent development of esophageal stricture. In 2020, the American Gastroenterology Association (AGA) and the Joint Task Force on Allergy-Immunology Practice Parameters (JTF) recommended certain guidelines on the management of EoE [32]. Currently, drugs, diet and dilation are the three main modalities of treatment of EoE.

12. Drugs

12.1 PPI

PPI is now used as the first-line treatment of EoE. In adults patients treated with PPI, symptomatic improvement can range from 25–80% and histological remission from 33–61% [33]. As mentioned before, PPI can block IL-4 stimulated eotaxin-3 secretion and thus can inhibit eosinophil recruitment from blood into the esophageal tissue [34]. Significant improvement of dysphagia can occur in few days' time. PPI can also be used as an adjunctive therapy when patients with EoE require esophageal dilation. Richter et al. found that esophageal eosinophilia was decreased in patients who received combination of PPI and esophageal dilation but not in patients who had esophageal dilation alone [35]. Finally, PPI can also restore the esophageal mucosal barrier function in patients with EoE and thus can inhibit the entry of aeroallergens into the esophageal mucosa [36]. It is author's opinion that in endotype 1, full dose of PPI once a day or low dose PPI twice a day should be initiated. Patients should be evaluated for symptomatic/clinical response after 4 weeks. At that time, there will be 2 groups:

1. Non-responders or inadequate clinical responders: dose of the PPI should be doubled and the patient should be evaluated again after 4 weeks. If there is no improvement of clinical response after 4 weeks, alternate therapy should be considered.

2. Responders or adequate clinical responders: same dose of PPI should be continued for another 4 weeks. Then the dose of PPI should be lowered to maintain controlling patient's symptoms.

A recent study found that in endotype 2, continuation of PPI therapy for at least 12 weeks had greater chance of inducing remission of EoE whereas in endotype 3, there was less responsiveness to PPI therapy both in the beginning and in the long run [37].

12.2 Topical glucocorticosteroids

Have become the second line medications for the treatment of EoE. Fluticasone metered dose inhaler 880 microgram puffed directly into the mouth without breathing and then dry swallowed twice a day for 6 to 8 weeks has been found to be effective in reducing symptoms and esophageal eosinophilia in 50 to 80% of cases [38, 39]. Patients are advised not to take any food or drink or rinse their mouth for half an hour to prevent the medication from washing off the esophageal mucosa. The maximal anti-inflammatory effect is found in proximal esophagus. Oral viscous budesonide (OVB) 1 mg twice a day also decreases dysphagia and esophageal eosinophilia. OVB is easy to swallow, more mucoadherent and is made by mixing aqueous solution of budesonide (1 mg/2 mL) with the sugar substitute sucralose (5 g), chocolate syrup or honey [40]. Both forms of topical corticosteroids are more effective in histologic improvement than symptomatic improvement. Only 1% of the topical steroid is absorbed, so systemic side effects are extremely rare although oral and esophageal candidiasis can occur in up to one third of the time and herpes simplex esophagitis have been reported rarely.

Topical steroid is generally given for 8 weeks. If that fails, prolonged or higher doses of topical steroids or systemic steroids or dietary treatment or esophageal dilation should be tried to get symptomatic improvement. The AGA/JTF suggests continuation of topical glucocortisteroids as maintenance therapy in patients with EoE in remission after short-term use of topical glucocoticosteroids.

13. Diet

Dietary therapy is very effective in the management of EoE. It can be used as an initial therapy or when other modalities of treatments fail. Dietary therapy depends on the resources available and can be expensive. As the dietary food allergen is removed, dietary therapy is very effective in inducing and maintaining clinicopathological remission. The three ways of dietary modification include:

1. Elemental diet: Amino acid based formula to remove food allergens. This therapy when given for a minimum of 6 weeks did both symptomatic and histologic improvement (95% and 98% respectively) in EoE patients [41]. But the amino acid formula is expensive and unpalatable which affect patients' quality of life, especially in children.

2. Sixfood group elimination diet (SFGED): The most common food allergens in EoE include milk, egg, wheat, soy, peanuts/tree nuts and sea food (fish/shellfish). Significant clinical and histological (74%) improvement occurred in EoE patients (children) when they were on this SFGED [42]. Another study showed fourfood group elimination diet (FFGED) which excludes milk, egg, wheat and legumes, when given for 6 weeks, clinicopathological remission occurred in 54% of adult EoE patient [43], and

3. Targeted or tailored elimination diet: This therapy is guided by detection of food allergens by skin prick/patch tests and blood tests. These tests can be not only time consuming but also can give false positive and false negative results. This therapy is offered as per the preference of the patient. Sixty-eight percent of EoE patients had symptomatic improvement on targeted therapy [44]. A dietitian interested in food allergies and EoE should be consulted. An Allergist should also be involved to find out the allergens triggering EoE. Food challenge by introducing one food or food group every 4 to 6 weeks should be offered. If the patient is allergic to food, there will be recurrence of symptoms and esophageal eosinophilia [45]. The AGA/JTF suggests using elemental diet or SFGED or testing based elimination diet over no treatment.

14. Systemic steroids

Oral methylprednisolone induced marked clinical and histological improvement in pediatric EoE patients [46]. Because of systemic side effects, this therapy is reserved when other therapeutic interventions fail. Steroids work by reducing the synthesis of eota xin3, IL5 and GMCSF, and inducing the apoptosis of eosinophils. But recurrence of the EoE occurs after withdrawal of the steroids. The AGA/JTF suggests topical glucocorticosteroids rather than systemic steroids should be used in patients with EoE.

15. Immunomodulators

Azathiopurine and 6mercaptopurine induced and maintained clinical and histological remission in steroid dependent EoE patients in a case series [47]. They are not currently recommended for routine clinical use in EoE.

16. Mast cell stabilizers

In a small case series, Cromolyn sodium failed to show any clinical or histologic improvement in EoE patients [48].

17. Leukotriene inhibitors

Montelukast is an eosinophil stabilizing agent. It improved clinical symptoms in EoE but there was no histological improvement [49].

17.1 IL-4 inhibitor

Dupilumab is an interleukin-4 receptor antagonist/monoclonal antibody. It has been found to be effective in improving dysphagia and esophageal eosinophilia (intraepithelial eosinophil count of ≤6 eosinophils per high-power field) in a double blind, placebo-controlled, pivotal phase 3 trial (Part A) that evaluated its efficacy in 81 patients aged ≥12 years with EoE. Dupilumab was granted Breakthrough Therapy designation by the FDA (Food and Drug Administration, USA) in September, 2020 for the treatment of the patients aged ≥12 years with EoE [50]. This designation would allow expedited review of dupilumab for the FDA approval.

17.2 IL-13 inhibitor

RPC4046 (a humanized monoclonal antibody against IL13) was found to improve dysphagia, and reduce histologic and endoscopic features compared with placebo in a phase II trial. The medication was also found to be safe and well tolerated [51].

17.3 IL-5 inhibitor

AntiIL5 antibody has been studied in both pediatric and adult patients with EoE. Mepolizumab significantly reduced esophageal eosinophilia but there was minimum symptomatic improvement [52]. Reslizumab also improved esophageal eosinophilia in EoE but there was no difference in clinical improvement in comparison to placebo [53, 54].

17.4 Macrophage migration inhibitory factor (MIF)

Macrophage migration inhibitory factor (MIF) is overexpressed in the esophageal mucosa of EoE patients. Recently, in the mice model of EoE, early administration a drug that blocked the action of MIF prevented eosinophilic infiltration in the esophagus. This study can lead to a novel therapy in future if MIF effect can be blocked in EoE patients [55].

The medications investigated for the treatment of EoE can be grouped as follows:

- Medications with proven effectiveness: PPI, topical glucocorticoids, systemic steroids. Immunomodulators.
- Medications under development: IL-4 inhibitor, IL-13 inhibitor, MIF.
- Medications with proven ineffectiveness: mast cell stabilizers, leukotriene inhibitors, IL-5 inhibitors.

18. Endoscopic treatment

Esophageal dilation has definitive role in the management of EoE. Dilation is not indicated in patients with normal caliber esophagus and signs of inflammation during endoscopy [56]. It is very effective in symptomatic esophageal stricture (esophageal diameter < 10 mm), long segment narrowing and narrow caliber esophagus. This modality of treatment improves dysphagia and quality of life but does not reduce esophageal eosinophilia [57]. Either hydrostatic balloon dilation or wire guided bougie dilation can be done. Esophageal diameter should be 15 to 18 mm to relieve dysphagia. Patients may need multiple sessions to achieve this. There is an increased risk of mucosal tear causing postdilation chest pain for several days [58]. Although initially thought that EoE patients carry higher risk of perforation after esophageal dilation, systematic review did not show any higher risk of perforation (0.1%) in this group of patients [59].

18.1 Endoscopic surveillance

Currently there is no guideline when surveillance endoscopy should be done in EoE patients who have achieved remission. In clinical practice, endoscopic and histologic assessment should be done 6 to 8 weeks after initiation or change of treatment to evaluate the efficacy of the treatment. When the disease is under remission, less frequent assessment/surveillance is done on a yearly basis or less frequently depending on the clinical scenario and the clinician.

18.2 Prognosis

As mentioned earlier, EoE is a chronic inflammatory disease of the esophagus. The inflammation leads to remodeling, fibrosis and stricture. Fortunately, no case of esophageal malignancy has been reported in EoE. Patients are generally diagnosed after several years of their symptoms. Although symptomatic improvement occurs after treatment, recurrence is common after discontinuation of treatment. So maintenance therapy is needed to prevent recurrences. At the present time there is no head to head study to suggest the best maintenance treatment. Continuation of PPI, swallowed glucocorticosteroid and/or dietary therapy should be done in all EoE patients particularly in those with history of food impaction, dysphagia, esophageal stricture, and in those with rapid symptomatic and histologic relapse following initial treatment.

19. Summary

EoE has become a common clinical entity in patients with dysphagia and esophageal food impaction. Although the disease is more common in young male patients with allergic disorders, any person can get affected. High degree of suspicion is essential to diagnose this disease. So multiple proximal and distal esophageal biopsies should be taken in EoE suggestive mucosa (EREFS) and even in normal looking mucosa. Other causes of esophageal eosinophilia particularly GERD, eosinophilic gastroenteritis and hypereosinophilic syndrome should be considered. The morbidity can be managed and long-term complications can be prevented by a multidisciplinary team which includes gastroenterologists, pathologists, allergists and dietitians. Patients with EoE should be given PPI therapy or topical glucocorticosteroids for 8 to 12 wk. If there is no clinicoopathological improvement i.e., in treatment-resistant cases, esophageal dilation should be offered [60]. Esophageal dilation in combination with PPI therapy or topical glucocorticosteroid therapy should be offered to patients with esophageal strictures and narrow caliber lumen. Lowest effective dose of PPI therapy or topical glucocorticosteroid should be continued to all EoE patients as maintenance therapy to reduce progression of the disease and relapse. Patients with EoE should be referred to the dietitians interested in food allergies and EoE patients. The AGA/JTF recommends using immunomodulators, IL-4 inhibitor or IL-13 inhibitor *only* in the context of clinical trial.

Conflict of interest

None.

Author contribution

Monjur Ahmed, MD, FRCP solely contributed to this work.

Author details

Monjur Ahmed
Thomas Jefferson University Hospital, Philadelphia, PA, USA

*Address all correspondence to: monjur.ahmed@jefferson.edu

References

[1] Park H. An overview of eosinophilic esophagitis. Gut Liver 2014; 8: 590-597 [PMID: 25368745 DOI: 10.5009/gnl14081].

[2] Attwood SEA, Smyrk TC, Demeester TR. Eosinophilic asthma-episodic dysphagia with eosinophilic infiltrates. Gut. 1989; 30:A1493

[3] Hruz P. Epidemiology of eosinophilic esophagitis. Dig Dis 2014; 32: 40-47 [PMID: 24603379 DOI: 10.1159/000357008]

[4] Dellon ES, Hirano I. Epidemiology and Natural History of Eosinophilic Esophagitis. Gastroenterology. 2018 Jan;154(2):319-332.e3. doi: 10.1053/j.gastro.2017.06.067. Epub 2017 Aug 1. PMID: 28774845; PMCID: PMC5794619.

[5] Raheem M, Leach ST, Day AS, Lemberg DA. The pathophysiology of eosinophilic esophagitis. Front Pediatr 2014; 2: 41 [PMID: 24910846 DOI: 10.3389/fped.2014.00041]

[6] Kottyan LC, Davis BP, Sherrill JD, Liu K, Rochman M, Kaufman K, Weirauch MT, Vaughn S, Lazaro S, Rupert AM, Kohram M, Stucke EM, Kemme KA, Magnusen A, He H, Dexheimer P, Chehade M, Wood RA, Pesek RD, Vickery BP, Fleischer DM, Lindbad R, Sampson HA, Mukkada VA, Putnam PE, Abonia JP, Martin LJ, Harley JB, Rothenberg ME. Genome-wide association analysis of eosinophilic esophagitis provides insight into the tissue specificity of this allergic disease. Nat Genet 2014; 46: 895-900 [PMID: 25017104 DOI: 10.1038/ng.3033]

[7] Spergel JM. New genetic links in eosinophilic esophagitis. Genome Med 2010; 2: 60 [PMID: 20822553 DOI: 10.1186/gm181]

[8] Malhotra N, Levine J. Eosinophilic esophagitis: an autoimmune esophageal disorder. Curr Probl Pediatr Adolesc Health Care 2014; 44: 335-340 [PMID: 25499460 DOI: 10.1016/j.cppeds.2014.10.004]

[9] Zhang X, Cheng E, Huo X, Yu C, Zhang Q, Pham TH, Wang DH, Spechler SJ, Souza RF. Omeprazole blocks STAT6 binding to the eotaxin-3 promoter in eosinophilic esophagitis cells. PLoS One 2012; 7: e50037 [PMID: 23185525 DOI: 10.1371/journal.pone.0050037]

[10] Alexander ES, Martin LJ, Collins MH, Kottyan LC, Sucharew H, He H, Mukkada VA, Succop PA, Abonia JP, Foote H, Eby MD, Grotjan TM, Greenler AJ, Dellon ES, Demain JG, Furuta GT, Gurian LE, Harley JB, Hopp RJ, Kagalwalla A, Kaul A, Nadeau KC, Noel RJ, Putnam PE, von Tiehl KF, Rothenberg ME. Twin and family studies reveal strong environmental and weaker genetic cues explaining heritability of eosinophilic esophagitis. J Allergy Clin Immunol 2014; 134: 1084-1092.e1 [PMID: 25258143 DOI: 10.1016/j.jaci.2014.07.021]

[11] Odze RD. Pathology of eosinophilic esophagitis: what the clinician needs to know. Am J Gastroenterol 2009; 104: 485-490 [PMID: 19174804 DOI: 10.1038/ajg.2008.40]

[12] Philpott H, Nandurkar S, Thien F, Gibson PR, Royce SG. Eosinophilic esophagitis: a clinicopathological review. Pharmacol Ther 2015; 146: 12-22 [PMID: 25200122 DOI: 10.1016/j.pharmthe ra.2014.09.001]

[13] Clayton F, Fang JC, Gleich GJ, Lucendo AJ, Olalla JM, Vinson LA, Lowichik A, Chen X, Emerson L, Cox K, O'Gorman MA, Peterson KA. Eosinophilic esophagitis in adults is associated with IgG4 and not mediated by IgE. Gastroenterology 2014; 147:

602-609 [PMID: 24907494 DOI: 10.1053/j.gastro.2014.05.036]

[14] Dellon ES. Diagnosis and management of eosinophilic esophagitis. Clin Gastroenterol Hepatol 2012; 10: 1066-1078 [PMID: 22728382 DOI: 10.1016/j.cgh.2012.06.003]

[15] Parfitt JR, Gregor JC, Suskin NG, Jawa HA, Driman DK. Eosinophilic esophagitis in adults: distinguishing features from gastroesophageal reflux disease: a study of 41 patients. Mod Pathol 2006; 19: 90-96 [PMID: 16258505 DOI: 10.1038/modpathol.3800498]

[16] Akyüz U, Akyüz F, Ozdil K, Altun H, Ağan AF, Ağan A. Food impaction in older age: Think about an eosinophilic esophagitis. World J Gastrointest Endosc 2013; 5: 79-80 [PMID: 23422854 DOI: 10.4253/wjge.v5.i2.79]

[17] Sperry SL, Crockett SD, Miller CB, Shaheen NJ, Dellon ES. Esophageal foreign-body impactions: epidemiology, time trends, and the impact of the increasing prevalence of eosinophilic esophagitis. Gastrointest Endosc 2011; 74: 985-991 [PMID: 21889135 DOI: 10.1016/j.gie.2011.06.029]

[18] Lynch KL, Dhalla S, Chedid V, Ravich WJ, Stein EM, Montgomery EA, Bochner BS, Clarke JO. Gender is a determinative factor in the initial clinical presentation of eosinophilic esophagitis. Dis Esophagus 2016; 29: 174-178 [PMID: 25626069 DOI: 10.1111/dote.12307]

[19] Vernon N, Mohananey D, Ghetmiri E, Ghaffari G. Esophageal rupture as a primary manifestation in eosinophilic esophagitis. *Case Rep Med* 2014; 2014: 673189 [PMID: 24899902 DOI: 10.1155/2014/673189]

[20] Moawad FJ, Veerappan GR, Lake JM, Maydonovitch CL, Haymore BR, Kosisky SE, Wong RK. Correlation between eosinophilic oesophagitis and aeroallergens. Aliment Pharmacol Ther 2010; 31: 509-515 [PMID: 19925501 DOI: 10.1111/j.1365-2036.2009.04199.

[21] Elias MK, Kopacova J, Arora AS, Dierkhising RA, Enders FT, Katzka DA, Kryzer LA, Halland M, Smyrk TC, Talley NJ, Alexander JA. The diagnosis of esophageal eosinophilia is not increased in the summer months. Dysphagia 2015; 30: 67-73 [PMID: 25288197 DOI: 10.1007/s00455-014-9574-1]

[22] Konikoff MR, Blanchard C, Kirby C, Buckmeier BK, Cohen MB, Heubi JE, Putnam PE, Rothenberg ME. Potential of blood eosinophils, eosinophil-derived neurotoxin, and eotaxin-3 as biomarkers of eosinophilic esophagitis. Clin Gastroenterol Hepatol 2006; 4: 1328-1336 [DOI: 10.1016/j.cgh.2006.08.013]

[23] Bondar RL, Stein F, Kassam MS, Dunphy PT, Bennett BS, Johnston KW. Cerebral blood flow velocities by transcranial Doppler during parabolic flight. J Clin Pharmacol 1991; 31: 915-919 [PMID: 1761720 DOI: 10.1111/j.1572-0241.2007.01396.x] 10.1111/j.1572-0241.2007.01396.x]

[24] Hirano I. Role of advanced diagnostics for eosinophilic esophagitis. Dig Dis 2014; 32: 78-83 [PMID: 24603385 DOI: 10.1159/000357014]

[25] Nurko S, Furuta GT. Eosinophilic esophagitis. Available from: URL: http//www.nature.com/gimo/contents/pt1/full/gimo49.html

[26] Dellon ES, Gebhart JH, Higgins LL, Hathorn KE, Woosley JT, Shaheen NJ. The esophageal biopsy "pull" sign: a highly specific and treatment-responsive endoscopic finding in eosinophilic esophagitis (with video). Gastrointest Endosc 2016; 83: 92-100

[PMID: 26142556 DOI: 10.1016/j.gie.2015.05.046].

[27] Nurko S, Rosen R, Furuta GT. Esophageal dysmotility in children with eosinophilic esophagitis: a study using prolonged esophageal manometry. Am J Gastroenterol 2009; 104: 3050-3057 [PMID: 19755968 DOI: 10.1038/ajg.2009.543]

[28] Fox VL, Nurko S, Teitelbaum JE, Badizadegan K, Furuta GT. High-resolution EUS in children with eosinophilic "allergic" esophagitis. Gastrointest Endosc 2003; 57: 30-36 [PMID: 12518127 DOI: 10.1067/mge.2003.33]

[29] Shoda T, Wen T, Aceves SS, Abonia JP, Atkins D, Bonis PA, Caldwell JM, Capocelli KE, Carpenter CL, Collins MH, Dellon ES, Eby MD, Gonsalves N, Gupta SK, Falk GW, Hirano I, Menard-Katcher P, Kuhl JT, Krischer JP, Leung J, Mukkada VA, Spergel JM, Trimarchi MP, Yang GY, Zimmermann N, Furuta GT, Rothenberg ME; Consortium of Eosinophilic Gastrointestinal Disease Researchers (CEGIR). Eosinophilic oesophagitis endotype classification by molecular, clinical, and histopathological analyses: a cross-sectional study. Lancet Gastroenterol Hepatol. 2018 Jul;3(7):477-488. doi: 10.1016/S2468-1253(18)30096-7. Epub 2018 May 3. PMID: 29730081; PMCID: PMC5997568.

[30] Dellon ES, Liacouras CA, Molina-Infante J, Furuta GT, Spergel JM, Zevit N, Spechler SJ, Attwood SE, Straumann A, Aceves SS, Alexander JA, Atkins D, Arva NC, Blanchard C, Bonis PA, Book WM, Capocelli KE, Chehade M, Cheng E, Collins MH, Davis CM, Dias JA, Di Lorenzo C, Dohil R, Dupont C, Falk GW, Ferreira CT, Fox A, Gonsalves NP, Gupta SK, Katzka DA, Kinoshita Y, Menard-Katcher C, Kodroff E, Metz DC, Miehlke S, Muir AB, Mukkada VA, Murch S, Nurko S, Ohtsuka Y, Orel R, Papadopoulou A, Peterson KA, Philpott H, Putnam PE, Richter JE, Rosen R, Rothenberg ME, Schoepfer A, Scott MM, Shah N, Sheikh J, Souza RF, Strobel MJ, Talley NJ, Vaezi MF, Vandenplas Y, Vieira MC, Walker MM, Wechsler JB, Wershil BK, Wen T, Yang GY, Hirano I, Bredenoord AJ. Updated International Consensus Diagnostic Criteria for Eosinophilic Esophagitis: Proceedings of the AGREE Conference. Gastroenterology. 2018 Oct;155(4):1022-1033.e10. doi: 10.1053/j.gastro.2018.07.009. Epub 2018 Sep 6. PMID: 30009819; PMCID: PMC6174113.

[31] Dellon ES, Gonsalves N, Hirano I, Furuta GT, Liacouras CA, Katzka DA; American College of Gastroenterology. ACG clinical guideline: Evidenced based approach to the diagnosis and management of esophageal eosinophilia and eosinophilic esophagitis (EoE). Am J Gastroenterol. 2013 May;108(5):679-692; quiz 693. doi: 10.1038/ajg.2013.71. Epub 2013 Apr 9. PMID: 23567357.

[32] Hirano I, Chan ES, Rank MA, Sharaf RN, Stollman NH, Stukus DR, Wang K, Greenhawt M, Falck-Ytter YT; AGA Institute Clinical Guidelines Committee; Joint Task Force on Allergy-Immunology Practice Parameters. AGA Institute and the Joint Task Force on Allergy-Immunology Practice Parameters Clinical Guidelines for the Management of Eosinophilic Esophagitis. Gastroenterology. 2020 May;158(6):1776-1786. doi: 10.1053/j.gastro.2020.02.038. PMID: 32359562.

[33] Molina-Infante J, Katzka DA, Gisbert JP. Review article: proton pump inhibitor therapy for suspected eosinophilic oesophagitis. Aliment Pharmacol Ther. 2013

Jun;37(12):1157-1164. doi: 10.1111/apt.12332. Epub 2013 May 8. PMID: 23656497.

[34] Cortes JR, Rivas MD, Molina-Infante J, Gonzalez-Nuñez MA, Perez-G M, Masa JF, Sanchez JF, Zamorano J. Omeprazole inhibits IL-4 and IL-13 signaling signal transducer and activator of transcription 6 activation and reduces lung inflammation in murine asthma. J Allergy Clin Immunol. 2009 Sep;124(3):607-10, 610.e1. doi: 10.1016/j.jaci.2009.06.023. Epub 2009 Aug 8. PMID: 19665777.

[35] Bohm ME, Richter JE. Review article: oesophageal dilation in adults with eosinophilic oesophagitis. Aliment Pharmacol Ther. 2011 Apr;33(7):748-757. doi: 10.1111/j.1365-2036.2011.04593.x. Epub 2011 Feb 14. PMID: 21320137.

[36] van Rhijn BD, Weijenborg PW, Verheij J, et al. Acid suppression restores impaired esophageal mucosal integrity in patients with esophageal eosinophilia. Gastmentenolrogy. 2013;144(5):S155.

[37] Laserna-Mendieta EJ, Casabona S, Guagnozzi D, Savarino E, Perelló A, Guardiola-Arévalo A, Barrio J, Pérez-Martínez I, Lund Krarup A, Alcedo J, de la Riva S, Rey-Iborra E, Santander C, Arias Á, Lucendo AJ; EUREOS EoE CONNECT Research group. Efficacy of proton pump inhibitor therapy for eosinophilic oesophagitis in 630 patients: results from the EoE connect registry. Aliment Pharmacol Ther. 2020 Sep;52(5):798-807. doi: 10.1111/apt.15957. Epub 2020 Jul 17. PMID: 32677040.

[38] Carr S, Watson W. Eosinophilic esophagitis. Allergy Asthma Clin Immunol 2011; 7 (Suppl 1): S8 [DOI: 10.1186/1710-1492-7-S1-S8].

[39] Remedios M, Campbell C, Jones DM, Kerlin P. Eosinophilic esophagitis in adults: clinical, endoscopic, histologic findings, and response to treatment with fluticasone propionate. Gastrointest Endosc 2006; 63: 3-12 [PMID: 16377308 DOI: 10.1016/j.gie.2005.07.049].

[40] Straumann A, Conus S, Degen L, Felder S, Kummer M, Engel H, Bussmann C, Beglinger C, Schoepfer A, Simon HU. Budesonide is effective in adolescent and adult patients with active eosinophilic esophagitis. Gastroenterology 2010; 139: 1526-1537, 1537.e1 [PMID: 20682320 DOI: 10.1053/j.gastro.2010.07.048]

[41] Kelly KJ, Lazenby AJ, Rowe PC, Yardley JH, Perman JA, Sampson HA. Eosinophilic esophagitis attributed to gastroesophageal reflux: improvement with an amino acid-based formula. Gastroenterology 1995; 109: 1503-1512 [PMID: 7557132 DOI: 10.1016/0016-5085(9 5)90637-1]

[42] Kagalwalla AF, Sentongo TA, Ritz S, Hess T, Nelson SP, Emerick KM, Melin-Aldana H, Li BU. Effect of six-food elimination diet on clinical and histologic outcomes in eosinophilic esophagitis. Clin Gastroenterol Hepatol 2006; 4: 1097-1102 [PMID: 16860614 DOI: 10.1016/j.cgh.2006.05.026]

[43] Molina-Infante J, Arias A, Barrio J, Rodríguez-Sánchez J, Sanchez-Cazalilla M, Lucendo AJ. Four-food group elimination diet for adult eosinophilic esophagitis: A prospective multicenter study. J Allergy Clin Immunol 2014; 134: 1093-1099.e1 [PMID: 25174868 DOI: 10.1016/j.jaci.2014.07.023]

[44] Wolf WA, Jerath MR, Sperry SL, Shaheen NJ, Dellon ES. Dietary elimination therapy is an effective option for adults with eosinophilic esophagitis. Clin Gastroenterol Hepatol

2014; 12: 1272-1279 [PMID: 24440337 DOI: 10.1016/j.cgh.2013.12.034]

[45] Gonsalves N, Yang GY, Doerfler B, Ritz S, Ditto AM, Hirano I. Elimination diet effectively treats eosinophilic esophagitis in adults; food reintroduction identifies causative factors. *Gastroenterology* 2012; 142: 1451-1459.e1; quiz e14- e15 [PMID: 22391333 DOI:

[46] Liacouras CA, Wenner WJ, Brown K, Ruchelli E. Primary eosinophilic esophagitis in children: successful treatment with oral corticosteroids. J Pediatr Gastroenterol Nutr 1998; 26: 380-385 [PMID: 9552132 DOI: 10.1097/00005176-199804000-00004]

[47] Netzer P, Gschossmann JM, Straumann A, Sendensky A, Weimann R, Schoepfer AM. Corticosteroid-dependent eosinophilic oesophagitis: azathioprine and 6-mercaptopurine can induce and maintain long-term remission. Eur J Gastroenterol Hepatol 2007; 19: 865-869 [PMID: 17873610 DOI: 10.1097/MEG.0b013e32825a6ab4]

[48] Liacouras CA, Spergel JM, Ruchelli E, Verma R, Mascarenhas M, Semeao E. Eosinophilic Esophagitis: A 10-Year Experience in 381 Children. Clin Gastroenterol Hepatol 2005; 3: 1198-1206 [DOI: 10.1016/S1542-3565(05)00885-2]

[49] Attwood SE, Lewis CJ, Bronder CS, Morris CD, Armstrong GR, Whittam J. Eosinophilic oesophagitis: a novel treatment using Montelukast. Gut 2003; 52: 181-185 [PMID: 12524397 DOI: 10.1136/gut.52.2.181]

[50] FDA grants Dupixent® (dupilumab) Breakthrough Therapy designation for eosinophilic esophagitis. https://www.prnewswire.com/news-releases/fda-grants-dupixent-dupilumab-breakthrough-therapy-designation-for-eosinophilic-esophagitis-301129713.html. Accessed September 14, 2020.

[51] Hirano I, Collins MH, Assouline-Dayan Y, Evans L, Gupta S, Schoepfer AM, Straumann A, Safroneeva E, Grimm M, Smith H, Tompkins CA, Woo A, Peach R, Frohna P, Gujrathi S, Penenberg DN, Li C, Opiteck GJ, Olson A, Aranda R, Rothenberg ME, Dellon ES; HEROES Study Group. RPC4046, a Monoclonal Antibody Against IL13, Reduces Histologic and Endoscopic Activity in Patients With Eosinophilic Esophagitis. Gastroenterology. 2019 Feb;156(3):592-603.e10. doi: 10.1053/j.gastro.2018.10.051. Epub 2018 Nov 2. PMID: 30395812.

[52] Straumann A, Conus S, Grzonka P, Kita H, Kephart G, Bussmann C, Beglinger C, Smith DA, Patel J, Byrne M, Simon HU. Anti-interleukin-5 antibody treatment (mepolizumab) in active eosinophilic oesophagitis: a randomised, placebo-controlled, double-blind trial. Gut. 2010 Jan;59(1):21-30. doi: 10.1136/gut.2009.178558. PMID: 19828470.

[53] Spergel JM, Rothenberg ME, Collins MH, Furuta GT, Markowitz JE, Fuchs G, O'Gorman MA, Abonia JP, Young J, Henkel T, Wilkins HJ, Liacouras CA. Reslizumab in children and adolescents with eosinophilic esophagitis: results of a double- blind, randomized, placebo-controlled trial. *J Allergy Clin Immunol* 2012; 129: 456-463, 463.e1-3 [PMID: 22206777 DOI: 10.1016/ j.jaci.2011.11.044]

[54] Assa'ad AH, Gupta SK, Collins MH, Thomson M, Heath AT, Smith DA, Perschy TL, Jurgensen CH, Ortega HG, Aceves SS. An antibody against IL-5 reduces numbers of esophageal intraepithelial eosinophils in children with eosinophilic esophagitis. Gastroenterology. 2011 Nov;141(5):1593-1604. doi: 10.1053/j.gastro.2011.07.044. Epub 2011 Aug 9. PMID: 21835135.

[55] de Souza HS, Tortori CA, Lintomen L, Figueiredo RT, Bernardazzi C, Leng L, Bucala R, Madi K, Buongusto F, Elia CC,

Castelo-Branco MT, Bozza MT. Macrophage migration inhibitory factor promotes eosinophil accumulation and tissue remodeling in eosinophilic esophagitis. Mucosal Immunol. 2015 Sep;8(5):1154-65. doi: 10.1038/mi.2015.6. Epub 2015 Feb 25. PMID: 25712805; PMCID: PMC4540676.

[56] Schoepfer A. Treatment of eosinophilic esophagitis by dilation. Dig Dis. 2014;32(1-2):130-133. doi: 10.1159/000357091. Epub 2014 Feb 28. PMID: 24603396.

[57] Schoepfer AM, Gonsalves N, Bussmann C, Conus S, Simon HU, Straumann A, Hirano I. Esophageal dilation in eosinophilic esophagitis: effectiveness, safety, and impact on the underlying inflammation. Am J Gastroenterol 2010; 105: 1062-1070 [PMID: 19935783 DOI: 10.1038/ajg.2009.657]

[58] Bohm ME, Richter JE. Review article: oesophageal dilation in adults with eosinophilic oesophagitis. Aliment Pharmacol Ther 2011; 33: 748-757 [PMID: 21320137 DOI: 10.1111/j.1365-2036.2011.04593.x]

[59] Jacobs JW, Spechler SJ. A systematic review of the risk of perforation during esophageal dilation for patients with eosinophilic esophagitis. Dig Dis Sci 2010; 55: 1512-1515 [PMID: 20238250 DOI: 10.1007/s10620-010-1165-x]

[60] Moole H, Jacob K, Duvvuri A, Moole V, Dharmapuri S, Boddireddy R, Uppu A, Puli SR. Role of endoscopic esophageal dilation in managing eosinophilic esophagitis: A systematic review and meta-analysis. Medicine (Baltimore). 2017 Apr;96(14):e5877. doi: 10.1097/MD.0000000000005877. PMID: 28383396; PMCID: PMC5411180.

Chapter 4

Extraesophageal Manifestations and Symptoms of Esophageal Diseases

Ljiljana Širić, Marinela Rosso and Aleksandar Včev

Abstract

Esophageal diseases are diagnosed by gastroenterological processing indicated due to typical gastrointestinal symptoms, but typical gastrointestinal symptoms are not the only possible manifestation of esophageal disease. There are also external symptoms such as chronic cough, laryngitis, pharyngitis, oropharyngeal dysphagia, odynophagia, laryngopharyngeal reflux, dysphonia, sinusitis, ear pain, and changes in laryngopharyngeal mucosa (erythema, edema, ventricular obliteration, cricoid hyperplasia and pseudosulcus). Extraesophageal symptoms are common in esophagitis and GERD, and studies show increasing prevalence of LPR in patients with GERD, as well as an association of reflux disease with cough and dysphonia symptoms. The aim of the chapter is to describe these extraesophageal symptoms of esophageal disease and how to recognize and treat them, in order to facilitate gastroenterologists' diagnostic processing of patients with these symptoms, improve their treatment and assessment of the therapy effectiveness, prevent the development of stronger symptoms, and encourage multidisciplinary cooperation and exchange of knowledge, scientific and clinical work.

Keywords: chronic cough, chronic laryngitis, dysphonia, esophagitis, laryngopharyngeal reflux

1. Introduction

Due to anatomical location and function, esophageal motility disorders, inflammatory diseases, gastroesophageal reflux (GER), esophageal rings and webs, tumors and other esophageal conditions and diseases can cause many extraesophageal symptoms, which are increasingly recognised and diagnosed by otolaryngologists, pulmonologists, cardiologists, and, of course, gastroenterologists. Certain pathophysiological conditions that are not localized in the esophagus may be the first symptoms of esophageal disease or signs associated with the onset of esophageal disease. One of the etiological factors is the pathophysiological mechanism of the increase in intra-abdominal pressure that occurs during weight gain and in pregnancy. Another etiological factor is the pathophysiological mechanism of relaxation of the lower esophageal sphincter that may occur due to coronary heart disease drug therapy rich in nitrates. A similar thing happens during antirheumatic therapy in rheumatoid arthritis and some degenerative

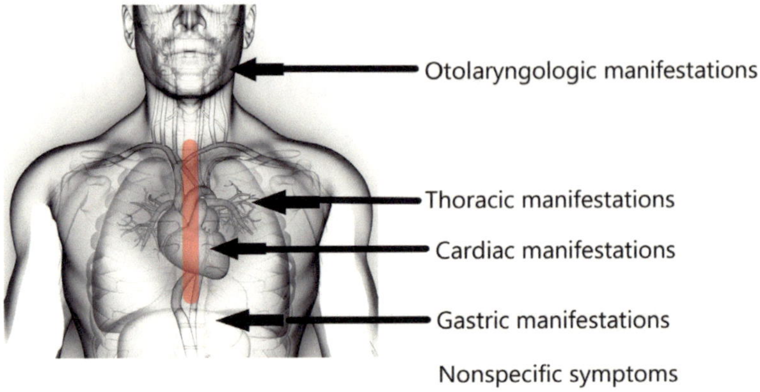

Figure 1.
Extraesophageal manifestation of esophageal diseases.

diseases of the locomotor system. Other conditions that may be associated with gastroesophageal reflux and esophageal diseases include diabetes mellitus, which results in prolonged gastric stagnation and consequent prolonged gastric emptying, and duodenal ulcer, duodenal stenosis, or malignant gastric disease in which delayed gastric emptying is present. So far, it is a well-known fact that the appropriate speed of food passage through the gastrointestinal tract, which is conditioned by a series of autoregulatory processes, is important. An optimal rate of passage is required - small enough to complete food digestion and absorption of substances and large enough to supply the body with the necessary nutrients in a timely manner [1]. The most common atypical symptoms of esophageal disease, primarily esophagitis and gastroesophageal reflux disease (GERD), will be listed here. For better visibility and easier understanding, the classification of atypical extraesophageal symptoms was performed according to the criterion of anatomical localization (**Figure 1**):

- otolaryngological manifestations
- thoracic manifestations
- cardiac manifestations

And last but not least, the biopsychosocial dimensions of esophageal diseases and extraesophageal symptoms are being recognized, too.

2. Otolaryngologic manifestations

2.1 Chronic laryngitis and laryngopharyngeal reflux (LPR)

Patients with reflux laryngitis often have characteristic anamnestic data and records in the history of the disease. Common symptoms of laryngitis include chronic or intermittent recurrent cough, chronic sore throat, hoarseness, clearing of the throat, dry mouth, feeling of a 'lump' and tickling in the throat, nocturnal dyspnea, laryngospasm and dyspepsia. Inspection of the laryngeal mucosa may reveal erythema and edema of the mucosa covering the arytenoid cartilage, the posterior part of the larynx, and often the posterior part of the true vocal cords.

Two theories explain the pathogenesis of reflux laryngitis:

1. theory of direct injury of the laryngeal mucosa and surrounding tissue by acid and pepsin;

2. reflex theory [2].

Due to direct injury to the laryngeal and pharyngeal mucosa, mucociliary transport is damaged and secretions accumulate in the throat, which causes additional irritation of the mucosa and contributes to the symptoms of postnasal drip, throat clearing and foreign body sensation in the throat. As the larynx lacks the protective external cleansing and salivary mechanisms that neutralize acid, gastric reflux remains undiluted for a long time, resulting in tissue injury. The action of pepsin leads to the depletion of the carbonic anhydrase isoenzyme III, and it catalyzes the reversible hydration of carbon dioxide resulting in the production of bicarbonate ions. The formation of bicarbonate ions directly neutralizes the acidic stomach contents and inactivates pepsin, so the ions actually protect the tissue from acid refluxate [3, 4]. On the other hand, depletion of carbonic anhydrase isoenzyme III reduces the neutralization of acidic gastric contents and allows its prolonged activity. According to the reflex theory, laryngopharyngeal reflux occurs due to esophageal reflux that stimulates vagal-mediated reflexes, resulting in a subjective need to 'clear' the throat and a chronic cough that leads to injury to the laryngeal mucosa. Laryngopharyngeal reflux is a clinical entity that represents the return of gastric contents to the space of the larynx and hypopharynx, which causes the contact of acid with the tissues of the upper aerodigestive tract [5]. In the physiological state, the upper and lower esophageal sphincters act together and prevent reflux of gastric contents into the esophagus and upper aerodigestive tract. However, the pathophysiology of LPR is typically attributed to a defect or dysfunction of the upper esophageal sphincter. The esophagus features a number of protective mechanisms which prevent injury of the mucosa, which the laryngopharyngeal mucosa do not possess, and are more susceptible to damage from acid reflux. Laryngeal epithelium is up to 100 times more susceptible to pepsin damage than esophageal tissue [6]. Regurgitation of the contents may cause primary burning and/or sore throat, cough, need for excessive throat cleansing, and secondarily may cause symptoms such as dysphonia, productive expectoration and globus hystericus (feeling of a 'lump' in the throat). Signs of laryngopharyngeal reflux are visible in the form of laryngeal irritations, hyperemic mucosa of the vocal cords and arytenoids, thinned vocal cords, posterior pharyngeal wall abnormalities, erythema, edema, and discontinuity of mucosal continuity. Of these symptoms, laryngeal irritations and abnormalities of the posterior pharyngeal wall have a statistically significant prevalence in patients with reflux. It should be noted that these symptoms, in addition to esophagitis and gastroesophageal reflux disease, are also present in persons exposed to allergens and irritants and in postnasal drip syndrome. Most authors interpret laryngopharyngeal reflux as atypical gastroesophageal reflux, although some authors disagree with this interpretation given the different pathophysiology and symptomatology of these refluxes [7]. It is important to emphasize that the etiology of reflux in laryngopharyngeal and gastroesophageal reflux is not the same, just as the form and circumstances of occurrence are not quite the same. For example, laryngopharyngeal reflux occurs more often during the day in an upright position, while gastroesophageal reflux occurs in a horizontal position and at night, or during sleep. Different body composition of patients with laryngopharyngeal and gastroesophageal reflux [8] was also observed, and published studies show an association between increased body mass index (identified as obesity) and gastroesophageal reflux disease [9] and a statistically significant higher incidence of gastroesophageal reflux disease in patients with registered obesity. In contrast, increased body mass index is not statistically significant in patients suffering from laryngopharyngeal reflux [10, 11]. Reflux associated with laryngeal symptoms is verified by laryngoscopy and 24-hour pH monitoring. Patients with laryngopharyngeal reflux without alarming symptoms are treated empirically with proton pump inhibitors for one to two months. If this type of therapy is effective, according to individual needs, the therapy is extended to six months with the aim of complete healing of the laryngeal and pharyngeal mucosa.

2.2 Dysphonia

Chronic gastroesophageal reflux is an etiological factor that contributes to the manifestation of laryngeal symptoms, primarily hoarseness. In addition to hoarseness, laryngopharyngeal reflux and laryngitis may occur. Koufman et al. found that 78% of dysphonic patients have gastroesophageal reflux disease [12]. According to Vashana, acid reflux is especially common in singers. The author explains this statement in several facts: muscle activity due to a vocal technique that works against the lower esophageal sphincter; inadequate feeding and sleep dynamics; emotional components and exposure to stressors typical of this profession [13].

2.3 Chronic rhinosinusitis (CRS)

More recent studies has reported significant association between gastroesophageal reflux and chronic rhinosinusitis, but the nature of the association is still unknown. Gastroesophageal reflux disease can cause several upper airway symptoms and change the physiology of nasopharyngeal mucosa, while upper airway diseases might also exacerbate GERD symptoms [14]. This associaton can be explained by three physiological mechanisms: the direct effect of acid or acidic vapor in the nasal mucosa, a dysfunction of the autonomous nervous system and the presence of Helicobacter pylori. It is known that the direct contact of the acid with the nasopharyngeal mucosa results in mucosal edema, with reduction of the mucociliary clearance and obstruction of the sinusal ostium. The acid reflux is an uncommon event in the nasopharynx and occurs in only 5% of GERD patients. Autonomic dysfunction, in this case the increase of the vagal tonus, may partly account the hyper-reactivity of the airways to acid. The Heliobacter pylori has been identified in the esophagus, palatine and tonsils, saliva and teeth, and is not known how its presence can result in some abnormalities of this tissues. Retrospective studies describe an improvement of 69 to 89% of the nasosinusal symptoms after GER treatment. Despite this knowlege, it is still not possible to state that the gastroesophageal reflux is one of the leading risk factors to chronic rhinosinuitis, but it must be researched as an unchaining factor when there is no other evident etiology. Howewer, GER symptoms are very prevalent in patients with chronic rhinosinusitis [15].

2.4 Chronic otitis media (COM)

Chronic otitis media may lead to tympanic membrane perforation as a consequence of unresolved and resistant middle ear infection, blockage of the Eustachian tube, insufficiency of ciliary clearance, or an injury to the ear persisting more than 3 months. Various microorganisms are considered as etiologic agents in COM. Other predisposing factors may also play role in persistence of the disease. Many recent studies have shown a potential association between gastroesophageal reflux and otitis media chronica [16]. Gastroesophageal reflux can be an inflammatory cofactor and can result in upper respiratory tract disorders, including COM in pediatric and adult age group. Otitis media with effusion is the most common cause of hearing loss in children. The pathogenesis is multifactorial: infections, impaired immunologic status, allergic history, anatomical problems, familial predisposition and enviromental factors have role in pathogenesis. The angle and length of the Eustachian tube are more horizontal and shorter in infants than in adults, and may allow reflux of gastric contens from the nasopharynx into the middle ear. It can cause to lay the groundwork for mucociliary clearance dysfunction and bacterial infections. Some studies found pepsin concentrations in samples from middle ear effusions of up to 1000-fold greater in children who undergone myringotomy. It was suggested that the GER may be related to glue ear in children. The therapy of COM is mainly surgical. Higher level of damage in the middle ear of patients having GERD requires appropriate treatment which may positively affect outcomes for COM surgery [17].

2.5 Oral mucosal changes

More recent studies have pointed out that extraesophageal symptoms of GERD are acidic lesions of the oral mucosa. These lesions are caused by direct acid and pepsin exposure, or acidic vapor contact in the oral cavity. GERD was reported to be associated with microscopic alterations in the palatal mucosa, such as epithelial atrophy, deepening of epithelial crests in connective tissue and a higher prevalence of fibroblasts [18]. Mucosal changes are quite common and not pathognomonic and specific of patients with gastroesophageal or esophagopharyngeal reflux, but erythema of the soft palate and uvula, epithelial atrophy, xerostomia and glositis are quite common in GERD patients. Some authors pointed out the presence of aphtoid lesions, hoarseness, chronic periodontitis, dry oral mucosa with a keratotic appearance of the gingival tissues and the presence of burning mouth. In addition, persons with GERD may complain of a sour or acidic taste, impaired taste (dysgeusia), an oral burning sensation and water brash (flooding of the mouth with saliva in response to an esophageal reflux stimulus) [19]. Adequate mucin-rich salivary secretions coat all of the internal anatomical surfaces and are essential for the protection of the oropharyngeal and esophageal mucosa and the teeth from chemical, thermal, mechanical and microbial damage. Saliva also facilitates efficient swallowing and speech. Some studies have found a significant association between gastroesophageal reflux and hyposalivation. On the other hand, proton pump inhibitors can cause hyposalivation. Hyposalivation may result in xerostomia, impaired mastication and swallowing, painful mouth, cracked lips and angular cheilitis [20].

2.6 Hypersalivation

The quantity of salivation and the quality of saliva can be an indicator of a certain disease of the oropharynx and esophagus or it can be an indicator of the complication of such conditions. Saliva is produced by the parotid, submandibular and sublingual glands and the small salivary glands. Sialoreia usually occurs in neurological diseases, such as Parkinson's and Wilson's disease, Angelman's syndrome, infections, heavy metal poisoning, and can also occur in the secretory phase of the menstrual cycle or as idiopathic paroxysmal sialoreia. Increased salivation can be caused by systemic consumption of drugs with a cholinergic effect (clozapine, risperidone, nitrazepam, lithium and bethanekol), and it also occurs as a subtle manifestation of gastroesophageal reflux disease in the form of 'water brash'. However, hypersalivation, although uncomfortable and disruptive, does not necessarily have to be negative since saliva plays an important role in protecting the esophageal mucosa. There are studies on the importance of ingested saliva that neutralizes the pH of gastric acid regurgitated into the esophagus [21] and on the buffering of gastric acid that enters the esophagus by reflux [22]. The acid that accumulates in the upper part of the esophagus reflexively initiates the formation of saliva [23], which is not the case when the acid accumulates in the lower part of the esophagus [24].

2.7 Dental erosion

Chronic regurgitation of gastric acids in patients with gastroesophageal reflux and related condition - laryngopharyngeal reflux may cause dental erosion which can, in combination with attrition or bruxism, lead to extensive loss of coronal tooth tissue. Dental erosion is typically a slowly-progressing and ireversibile phenomenon defined as the loss of tooth substance by chemical processes (acid exposure) not involving bacteria [25]. The literature shows a strong correlation between GERD and dental erosion, with a median prevalence of 24% in a large range of age groups. The degree of erosion due to GERD is related to the duration of the disease, frequency of reflux, the pH and type of acid, and the quality and quantity of saliva. Demineralisation and the loss of calcium and phosphate ions from the mineral surface of the teeth result in visible defects, and cause significant reduction in microhardness which makes the softened surface more prone to mechanical damage [26]. It is recognized that refluxed acid attacks the palatal surfaces of the upper incisor teeth first, later, if the condition continues, erosion of the occlusal surfaces of the posterior teeth in both arches and the labial or buccal surfaces [27].

2.8 Halitosis

Halitosis is an unpleasant odor from the oral cavity and is a condition that affects a large number of people [28]. The prevalence of halitosis is 8–46% [29]. The pathophysiological mechanism of halitosis is still not completely clear and is mainly attributed to oral pathology due to microbial activity in the interdental space, between the teeth and periodontium, and on the dorsal side of the tongue. Published data suggest that halitosis may correlate with chronic sinusitis, upper and lower respiratory tract diseases, various systemic diseases, gastroenterological diseases, and consumption of certain drugs in patients without oral pathology. It has been stated that mouth breathing, too, can be the cause of halitosis [30]. Although halitosis has previously been considered a rare consequence of gastrointestinal disorders [31], recent literal data have shown that it is common in gastrointestinal pathology and is significantly more common in patients with gastroesophageal reflux disease than in healthy individuals [32]. Furthermore, the symptom is often present in patients with verified infection with Helicobacter pylori, a bacterium that is among the major pathogenic factors of inflammatory and ulcerative changes on the gastric mucosa [33–36]. In addition, a high correlation has been demonstrated between halitosis and gastroesophageal reflux disease and peptic ulcer disease [37], and some authors have linked halitosis to volatile sulfur compounds [30, 38, 39] and to the chemical compounds cadaverine, some types of indoles [30]. Cadaverine (1,5-pentanediamine) is a toxic diamine formed by tissue putrefaction. Indole (benzopyrrole) is a heterocyclic compound formed by the breakdown of the amino acid tryptophan in the digestive tract, however, it is also used in the production of certain drugs, fragrances and essential oils [40]. An organic compound from the indole family associated with halitosis is skatol (3-methylindole), which occurs naturally in faeces, it is also present in flowers and essential oils (orange and jasmine) in low concentrations, and is used as a fixative in many perfumes [41]. A 2006 study by Lee et al. reported that Helicobacter pylori produces hydrogen sulfide and methyl mercaptan that contribute to halitosis [42], and the bacterium itself is one of the main factors in the manifestation of gastrointestinal diseases.

3. Thoracic manifestations

Thoracic manifestations can occur secondary to the wide range of esophageal disorders: inflammatory process, infections, trauma and perforation, congenital malformations, esophageal motility disorders and benign and malignant neoplasms. Complications associated with these diseases and disorders can involve the mediastinum, tracheobronchial tree, and lungs. Lower respiratory system and esophagus share a common embryological derivation and are anatomically related. Pulmonary complications can be associated with high morbidity and mortality. Such complications can be categorized as:

1. mediastinal complications (due to trauma, perforation, foreign bodies, caustic injury, or malignancy);

2. tracheobronchial complications (congenital or acquired tracheoesophageal fistulas);

3. pleural complications (esophagopleural fistulas);

4. lung complications (due to GERD, infectious and inflammatory process) [43].

Gastroesophageal reflux disease has been linked to a variety of respiratory diseases either as a direct cause, or as a risk factor to the inability to control or worsening of the disease. It can cause various pulmonary manifestations and nonspecific complaints: chronic cough and fewer, recurrent pneumonia, noncardiac chest pain, sputum production and dyspnoea, bronchospasm. Epidemiological studies in patients with reflux esophagitis have shown an increased risk for chronic bronchitis, chronic obstructive pulmonary disease, pneumonia, and idiopathic pulmonary fibrosis. Chronic cough and bronchial asthma are more common respiratory manifestations of GERD. Pathological GERD has been described in 30% to 80% of patients with asthma. Micro-aspiration of gastric contents and/or vagal irritation from gastro esophageal reflux may constitute airway irritants and thus represent a potential pathogenic mechanism for acute illness or acute exacerbations of chronic pulmonary diseases. Exacerbations of chronic obstructive pulmonary disease is twice as high in patients with GERD as in those without GERD symptoms. GERD can produce lung disease by two mechanisms: by reflex neural mechanisms occuring during reflux events limited to the lower part of esophagus, and direct from gastric contents refluxed into the pharynx producing upper airway damage and lung disease. While gastroesophageal reflux may increase airways resistance and cause inflammation by releasing pro-inflammatory mediators, esophagopharyngeal reflux creates the potential to aspiration and its consequences which varies depending of the duration, volume and nature of the aspirate [44]. Chronic cough is considered to be a cough that is continuously present for eight weeks and longer. Among the etiological factors, the three most common causes of chronic cough can be singled out: postnasal drip syndrome, asthma and gastroesophageal reflux. In 75% of cases, patients with chronic cough do not have the typical symptoms of esophagitis or gastroesophageal reflux disease, yet the result of 25% of patients with symptoms of both types speaks in favor of the association of chronic cough and esophageal disease [45]. Namely, the determination of correlation is primarily based on the strength and direction of the correlation, and not only on the frequency and percentage of results.

4. Cardiac manifestations

Coronary heart disease and gastroesophageal reflux disease can interact and produce chest pain. Some recent studies have shown that exposure of the esophageal mucosa to acid can compromise myocardial perfusion and cause chest pain by inducing coronary spasm or cardiac dysrythmia [46–48]. On the other hand, myocardial ischemia can cause esophageal dysmotility or relaxation of the lower esophageal sphincter and exacerbate GERD [49]. GERD can worsen sleep disturbances, and sleep apnea increases the risk of a cardiovascular diseases [50]. These two diseases have a number of common risk factors and comorbidities, such as diabetes, hypertension, hyperlipidemia, smoking and alcoholism, gender and age [51, 52]. Proton pump inhibitors, as a treatment option in GERD therapy can also affect cardiovascular physiology. One of the big population-based study shows that PPI usage can reduce the cardioprotective effects of certain therapies, and it can also reduce the contractility of myocardial tissue and raise the risk of atherosclerosis by increasing the serum levels of homocysteine by impairing the absorption of vitamin B12. This study indicates that GERD is associated with an increased risk of developing coronary heart disease, and PPI therapy that lasts longer than one year might increase the risk of CHD [53].

5. Conclusion

Esophageal symptoms are common and often overlap between different esophageal disorders, making a diagnosis based solely on patient history, symptoms, and physical presentation challenging. Esophageal motility disorders often manifest with chest pain and dysphagia. Other symptoms are heartburn, regurgitation, weight loss and malnutrition. Chest pain is localized behind the sternum, and does not spread to the shoulders and arms, which distinguishes it from cardiac pain. Gastroesophageal reflux (GER) symptoms have been reported in up to 20% of the adult population, which makes GER one of the common gastrointestinal disorders with a chronic or recurrent nature. Patients often complain of heartburn and acid regurgitation. The presence of this symptoms at least once a week for the last 3 months are considered essential in diagnosis of a clinical disorder called gastroesophageal reflux disease (GERD) [54]. Gastroesophageal reflux is often associated with symptoms of the respiratory tract. Chronic cough of unknown origin, laryngeal complaints, throat discomfort, breathing disorders, bronchitis, pneumonia and even non allergic asthma, resistant to steroid therapy, are suspicious of being reflux related. Other symptoms are haematemesis, eructation, dysphagia, odynophagia, hiccups, changes in the oral, nasal and pharyngeal mucosa, dental erosions and cardiac problems. Laryngopharyngeal reflux (LPR) is present in up to 60% of GERD patients. Symptoms of this multifactorial syndrome are mainly extraesophageal, and are found in the head and neck region. The most common symptoms are cough, hoarseness, dysphonia, sore throat, globus pharyngeus, chronic postnasal drip, and Eustachian tube dysfunction, Some studies have shown that LPR has been associated with vocal cord polyps, vocal cord granulomas, laryngospasm, subglottic stenosis and laryngeal carcinoma [55]. Esophagitis can be caused by reflux mechanism, infections, caustic agents, ionizing radiation, thermal injuries, eating disorders, medications, and as a part of some sistemic diseases. The most common symptoms are dysphagia and odynophagia, heartburn and acid regurgitation, haematemesis. Severe and prolonged vomiting and straining can results in tears in the mucous membrane of the esophagus. This condition is called Mallory-Weiss Syndrome. The main symptoms are hematemesis and melena, and in severe cases heavier bleeding may occur. Ribs and webs are the most common structural abnormalities of the esophagus. Most of them are asymptomatic, but can occasionally present with intermittent dysphagia to solids. They are associated with Zenker's diverticulum and Plummer-Vinson Syndrome which is classically a triad of dysphagia, iron-deficiency anemia, and esophageal webs. Esophageal rings are almost always associated with a hiatal hernia [56]. The esophagus is the most common site of acute foreign body obstruction. The clinical presentation varies from mild to extremely severe, and the most common symptoms are hypersalivation and odynophagia [57]. Esophageal perforation is a rare and potentially life-threatening condition most commonly caused by manipulations with medical instruments, forced strining and foreign bodies. The most common symptoms are odynophagia, chest pain, vomiting and shortness of breath, and in 70% of patients with perforation of the intrathoracic esophagus there are pleuromediastinum and palpable crepitus in the soft tissue of the neck and thorax. Caustic injuries of the esophagus are potentially one of the most challenging clinical situations in gastroenterology. Caustics and corrosives cause tissue injury by a chemical reaction. The severity of injury and the clinical presentation depends on several aspects: Concentration of the substance, amount ingested, duration of tissue contact, location of damage, and pH of the agent: hoarseness, stridor, dysphagia, odynophagia, hematemesis, epigastric pain. Short-term complications include perforation and death [58, 59]. Esophageal cancer is the sixth most common cause of cancer deaths worldwide. In the initial stage it usually shows no symptoms. The most common symptoms are dysphagia, chest pain, pressure or burning, heartburn, coughing or hoarseness, weight loss, bleeding, and hiccups. As can be seen, almost all esophageal diseases shows atypical and extraesophageal symptomatology. Due to proper and accurate diagnosis and treatment, the cooperation of a multidisciplinary team is required.

Acknowledgements

We would like to thank Ms. Mirna Brunčić for translating this text.

Conflict of interest

The authors have no conflict of interest.

Notes

The figure is from the author's own source.

Author details

Ljiljana Širić[1,2]*, Marinela Rosso[3] and Aleksandar Včev[4]

1 Department of Otorhinolaryngology, Head and Neck Surgery, University Hospital Center Osijek, Osijek, Croatia

2 Department of General and Applied Kinesiology, Faculty of Kinesiology, University of Zagreb, Zagreb, Croatia

3 Polyclinic Rosso, Osijek, Croatia

4 Faculty of Medicine, Faculty of Dental Medicine and Health, J.J. Strossmayer University of Osijek, Osijek, Croatia

*Address all correspondence to: ljsiric@gmail.com

References

[1] Guyton AC. Kretanje hrane kroz alimentarni trakt. In: Guyton AC. Medicinska fiziologija. Medicinska knjiga: Beograd - Zagreb, 1965., page 779.

[2] Toohill RJ, Kuhn JC. Role of refluxed acid in pathogenesis of laryngeal disorders. Am J Med. 1997;103(5A):100S–106S.

[3] Friedman M, Schalch P, Vidyasagar R, Kakodkar KA, Mazloom N, Joseph NJ. Wireless upper esophageal monitoring for laryngopharyngeal reflux (LPR). Otolaryngol Head Neck Surg. 2007;137(3):471-476.

[4] Weigt J, Mönkemüller K, Peitz U, Malfertheiner P. Multichannel intraluminal impedance and pH-metry for investigation of symptomatic gastroesophageal reflux disease. Dig Dis. 2007;25(3):179-182.

[5] Ford CN. Evaluation and management of laryngopharyngeal reflux. JAMA. 2005; 294:1534-1540.

[6] Koufman, JA. Laryngopharyngeal reflux is different from classic gastroesophageal reflux disease. Ear, Nose & Throat Journal. 2002;81(9):7-9.

[7] Koufman JA. Laryngopharyngeal reflux 2002: a new paradigm of airway disease. Ear Nose Throat J. 2002;81(9):S2–S6.

[8] Lim CH, Choi MG, Baeg MK i sur. Symptom Characteristics and Psychosomatic Proiles in Diferent Spectrum of Gastroesophageal Relfux Disease. Gut Liver 2014; 8: 165-169.

[9] Tan BK, Chandra RK,Pollak J i sur. Incidence and associated pre-morbid diagnoses of patients with chronic rhinosinusitis. J Allergy Clin Immunol 2013; 131: 1350-1360.

[10] Yilmaz T, Bajin MD, Gunaydin RO, Ozer S, Sozen T. Laryngopharyngeal rel ux and Helicobacter pylori. World J Gastroenterol 2014; 20: 8964-8970.

[11] Saruc M, Aksoy EA, Vardereli E i sur. Risk factors for laryngopharyngeal rel ux. Eur Arch Otorhinolaryngol 2012; 269: 1189-1194.

[12] Koufman JA, Wiener CJ, Wu WC, Castell DO. Reflux laryngitis and it's sequelae: The diagnostic role of ambulatory 24-hour pH monitoring. J Voice 1988;2(l):78-89.

[13] Vashani K, Murugesh M, Hattiangadi G, Gore G, Keer V, Ramesh VS, Sandur V, Bhatia SJ. Effectiveness of voice therapy in reflux-related voice disorders. Dis Esophagus. 2010 Jan;23(1):27-32.

[14] Coelho MS, Spolaor MR, Filho EDM, Sirena E, Romam P, Oliviera MSB, et al. Incidence of gastroesophageal reflux symptoms in patients with refractory chronic sinusitis upon clinical treatment. Int Arch Otorhinolaryngol. 2009;13(3):300-303.

[15] Loehrl TA, Smith TL. Chronic sinusitis and gastroesophageal reflux: are they related? Current Opinion in Otolaryngology & Head and Neck Surgery. 2004;12(1):18-20.

[16] Yazdi AK, Tajdini A, Malekzadeh R, Nasseri-Moghaddam S, Mazlum M, Nokhbeh-Zaeem H, Biazar P, Amiri M. Tretman of gastro-esophageal reflux disease may improve surgical outcomes for chronic otitis media. Middle East J Dig. Dis.2012;4(4);224-227.

[17] Yuksel F, Dogan M, Karatas D, Yuce S, Senturk M, Kulahli I. Clinical presentation of gastroesophageal reflux disease in children with chronic otitis media with effusion. J Craniofac Surg.2013;24(2):380-383.

[18] Silva MA, Damante JH, Stipp AC, Tolentino MM, Carlotto PR, Fleury RN. Gastroesophageal reflux disease: new oral findings. Oral Surg. Oral Med. Oral Pathol. Oral Radiol. Endod. 2001; 91: 301-310.

[19] Deppe H, Mucke T, Wagenpfeil S, Kesting M, Rozej A, Bajbouj M, Sculean A. Erosive esophageal reflux vs. non erosive esophageal reflu: oral findings in 71 patient. BMC Oral Health.2015;15:84.

[20] Ranjitkar S, Smales RJ, Kaidonis JA. Oral manifestations of gastroesophageal reflux disease. Journal of Gastroenterology and Hepatology.2012;27(1):21-27.

[21] Boyce HW, Bakheet MR. Sialorrhea: a review of a vexing, often unrecognized sign of oropharyngeal and esophageal disease. J Clin Gastroenterol. 2005 Feb;39(2):89-97.

[22] Burgess J. Salivary stimulation-could it play a role in GERD management? J Otolaryngol ENT Res. 2018;10(3):127-130.

[23] Shafik A, El-Sibai O, Shafik AA, etal. Effect of to picaleso phagealacidification on salivary secretion: identification of themechanism of action. J Gastroenterol Hepatol. 2005;20(12):1935-1939.

[24] Dutta SK, Agrawal K, Mahmoud MA. Modulation of salivation and heart burn in response to the site ofacidinfusioninthe human oesophagus. Aliment Pharmacol Ther. 2010;32(6):795-800.

[25] Lussi A. Erosive tooth wear - a multifactorial condition of growing concern and increasing knowledge. Monographs in Oral Scieence. 2006;20:1-8.

[26] Dundar A, Sengun A. Dental approach to erosive tooth wear in gastroesophageal reflux disease. Afr Health Sci.2014;14(2):481-486.

[27] Cengiz S, Cengiz MI, Saraç YS. Dental erosion caused by gastroesophageal reflux disease: a case report. Cases J. 2009;2:8018. doi:10.4076/1757-1626-2-8018.

[28] Alavi G, Alavi A, Saberfiroozi M, Sarbazi A, Motamedi M, Hamedani S. Dental erosion in patients with gastroesophageal reflux disease (GERD) in a sample of patients referred to the Motahari Clinic. J Dent (Shiraz). 2014; 15(1): 33-38.

[29] Kinberg S, Stein M, Zion N, Shaoul R. The gastrointestinal aspects of halitosis. Can J Gastroenterol. 2010;24(9):552-556.

[30] Iwanicka-Grzegorek E, Michalik J, Kepa J, Wierzbicka M, Aleksinski M, Pierzynowska E. Subjective patients' opinion and evaluation of halitosis using halimeter and organoleptic scores. Oral Dis. 2005;11(1):86-88.

[31] Warren JR, Marshall B. Unidentified curved bacilli on gastric epithelium in active chronic gastritis. Lancet. 1983;1:1273-1275.

[32] Sherman P, Czinn S, Drumm B, et al. Helicobacter pylori infection in children and adolescents: Working Group Report of the First World Congress of Pediatric Gastroenterology, Hepatology, and Nutrition. J Pediatr Gastroenterol Nutr. 2002;35(2):S128–S133.

[33] Di Fede O, Di Liberto C, Occhipinti G, et al. Oral manifestations in patients with gastro-oesophageal reflux disease: A single-center case-control study. J Oral Pathol Med. 2008;37:336-340.

[34] Suerbaum S, Michetti P. Helicobacter pylori infection. N Engl J Med. 2002;347:1175-1186.

[35] Katsinelos P, Tziomalos K, Chatzimavroudis G, et al. Eradication therapy in Helicobacter pylori-positive patients with halitosis: Long-term outcome. Med Princ Pract. 2007;16:119-123.

[36] Poelmans J, Feenstra L, Demedts I, Rutgeerts P, Tack J. The yield of upper gastrointestinal endoscopy in patients with suspected reflux-related chronic ear, nose, and throat symptoms. Am J Gastroenterol. 2004;99:1419-1426.

[37] Romano C, Cardile S. Gastroesophageal reflux disease and oral manifestation. Ital J Pediatr. 2014;40(1):A73.

[38] Moshkowitz M, Horowitz N, Leshno M, Halpern Z. Halitosis and gastroesophageal reflux disease: A possible association. Oral Dis. 2007;13:581-585.

[39] Izquierdo C, Gomez-Tamayo JC, Nebel JC, Pardo L, Gonzalez A. Identifying human diamine sensors for death related putrescine and cadaverine molecules. PLOS Computational Biology, 2018;14(1):e1005945.

[40] Atkins PW, De Paula J. Physical Chemistry. 8th ed. New York: W.H. Freeman, 2006.

[41] Li Q, Cheng T, Wang Y, Bryant SH .PubChem as a public resource for drug discovery. Drug Discov Today, 2010;15(23-24):1052-1057.

[42] Lee H, Kho HS, Chung JW, Chung SC, Kim YK. Volatile sulfur compounds produced by Helicobacter pylori. J Clin Gastroenterol. 2006;40:421-426.

[43] Giménez A, Franquet T, Erasmus JJ, Martínez S, Estrada P. Thoracic complications of esophageal disorders. Radiographics. 2002 Oct;22 Spec No:S247-58. doi: 10.1148/radiographics.22.suppl_1.g02oc18s247.

[44] Gaude GS. Pulmonary manifestations of gastroesophageal reflux disease. Ann Thorac Med.2009;4:115.23.

[45] Yuksel ES, Vaezi MF. Extraoseo phageal manifestations of gastrooesophageal reflux disease: cough, asthma, laryngitis, chest pain. Swiss Med Wkly 2012; 142. doi:10.4414/smw.2012.13544.

[46] Dent J, El-Serag HB, Wallander MA, et al. Epidemiology of gastro-oesophageal reflux disease: a systemic review. Gut 2005; 54:710-717.

[47] Chauhan A, Petch MC, Shofield PM. Effect of esophageal acid instillation on coronary artery blood flow. Lancet 1993; 341:1309-1310.

[48] Manisty C, Hughes-Roberts Y, Kaddoura S. Cardiac manifestations and sequelae of gastrointestinal disorders. Br J Cardiol 2009; 16:175-180.

[49] Liu Y, He S, Chen Y, et al. Acid reflux in patients with coronary artery disease and refractory chest pain. Intern Med 2013; 52:1165-1171.

[50] Fujiwara Y, Fass R. Gastroeso phageal reflux disease and sleep disturbances. J Gastroenterol 2012; 47:760-769.

[51] Chien KL, Hsu HC, Sung FC, et al. Metabolic syndrome as a risk factor for coronary artery disease and stroke: an 11-year prospective cohort in Taiwan community. Atherosclerosis 2007; 194:214-221.

[52] Okwuosa TM, Klein O, Chan C, et al. 13-Year long-term associations between changes in traditional cardiovascular risk factors and changes in fibrogen levels: the coronary artery risk development in young adults (CARDIA) study. Atherosclerosis 2013; 22:214-219.

[53] Chen CH, Lin CL, Kao CH. Association between gastroesophageal reflux disease and coronary heart disease: A nationwide population-based analysis. Medicine(Baltimore).2016;95(27):e4089.doi:10.1097/MD.0000000000004089. PMID: 27399102; PMCID: PMC5058831.

[54] Choi, J., Jung, H., Song, E., Shim, K., & Jung, S. Determinants of symptoms in gastroesophageal reflux disease: nonerosive reflux disease, symptomatic, and silent erosive reflux disease. European Journal of Gastroenterology & Hepatology, 2013;25(7):764-771.

[55] Hassan, WA. Laryngeal polyp associated with reflux disease: a case report. J Med Case Reports, 2020;14, 2.

[56] Ghazaleh S, Patel K. Esophageal Webs And Rings. [Internet]. 2020. Available from: https://www.ncbi.nlm.nih.gov/books/NBK539771/ [Accessed: 2020-12-29].

[57] Søreide JA, Viste A. Esophageal perforation: diagnostic work-up and clinical decision-making in the first 24 hours. Scand J Trauma Resusc Emerg Med. 2011;19:66. Published 2011 Oct 30. doi:10.1186/1757-7241-19-66.

[58] Katzka, D.A. Caustic injury to the esophagus. Curr Treat Options Gastro, 2001;4:59-66.

[59] De Lusong MAA, Timbol ABG, Tuazon DJS. Management of esophageal caustic injury. World J Gastrointest Pharmacol Ther. 2017;8(2):90-98.

Chapter 5

Introducing an Innovative Oral Neuromuscular Treatment of the Underlying Reason for Reflux Caused by Hiatus Hernia: An Aggravating Factor in Esophagitis

Mary Hägg and Thomas Franzén

Abstract

Esophagitis is a debilitating disease often leading to more serious conditions. It is aggravated by refluxed stomach acids for which the usual treatment is PPI drugs that at best treat the symptoms, not the underlying cause of reflux. Surgical interventions address the root - Hiatal muscular incompetence - but are invasive and expensive. Both treatments have proven unwanted side-effects. Neuromuscular treatment is a new and innovative alternative that addresses the root cause of reflux. The science and evidence behind this treatment is presented here. Reflux cannot happen when the diaphragm functions properly and maintains adequate pressure in the Hiatal canal, otherwise the neck of the stomach can intrude through the diaphragm into the chest cavity allowing reflux and conditions such as GERD, LPR, silent reflux, dyspepsia and more. This is especially common at night, when in bed. Training with a simple and inexpensive neuromuscular medical device takes 90 seconds per day, self-administered by the patient without medication or surgical intervention. No negative side effects are recorded for this treatment. Currently, 40 000 individuals have treated with the device. It is deployed in healthcare institutions in several countries and is recognised in the UK by NICE in a briefing to the NHS as a treatment for Hiatal hernia.

Keywords: dysphagia, esophagitis, GERD, hiatal hernia, hiatal incompetence, manometry, neuromuscular treatment, obesity, PPI medication, reflux

1. Introduction

Esophagitis is thoroughly explained as a condition elsewhere in this book and its various causes discussed. There can be a variety of causes of esophagitis but in all cases it is aggravated if Gastro Oesophageal Reflux Disease (GERD) is present. It is that condition, reflux that will be discussed here: its treatments, causes, similar conditions, and a new and innovative treatment that simply and effectively addresses the root cause of reflux – not just its symptoms. Damage caused by reflux to the lining of the oesophagus can lead to the condition of Barrett's oesophagus in which cell changes indicate a pre-cancerous condition [1, 2]. This chapter will

IntechOpen

explain what Hiatal hernia (HH) is and why it is near-exclusively [3, 4] responsible for all reflux-related conditions. It will be seen that the current most common active treatment for the symptoms of reflux is the administration of medication, often Proton Pump Inhibitor (PPI) drugs. These successfully alleviate the symptoms by reducing stomach acid production and its efficacy but, because they do not address the underlying cause of the condition, they are often prescribed for many years or even to end-of life. Their unwanted side-effects are well documented and referenced here. Medical science and healthcare professionals concerned with treating all symptoms caused by reflux should be excited and interested in a new, but proven, treatment that is simple, cheap, self-administered and with no negative side-effects. This disruptive technology to drug research and development is presented here.

2. Current treatments

In most cases clinicians first advise patients who present with reflux and the symptoms of reflux to implement lifestyle changes. These include changes in eating and drinking habits: lose weight, drink less alcohol, stop smoking, do not eat too close to bedtime, and more. Doctors also advise sleeping with the head of the bed raised, this encourages the neck of the stomach to remain correctly positioned and not intrude through the diaphragm at night allowing reflux. Changes in diet are often popular with patients with certain foods being excluded or included in their symptom-management routines.

The second, and most common type of treatment administered, is medication. This can be mild, over-the-counter (OTC) drugs, but is usually prescription drugs from the Proton Pump Inhibitor (PPI) class.

The third and last widely used type of intervention is surgery. Laparoscopic fundoplication is common, as are magnetic bands around the hiatal canal, and other operations. In essence each of these interventions is designed to compensate for the muscular incompetence in the diaphragm that allows the stomach neck to herniate into the chest cavity and reflux stomach contents.

2.1 Shortcomings of current treatments

Lifestyle changes are the most innocuous treatment and suffice for some people. Evidence [5] shows however, that their effect is weak.

Many OTC medications have a base pH and address the problem of reflux by reducing the acidity of the stomach acids which are being refluxed. Although the unpleasant sensations of reflux are reduced, the harmful effects on the vulnerable oesophagus and other organs continues. Long-term use of OTC medication is generally regarded to be free from harmful side-effects.

PPI medications act by inhibiting the amount and strength of the acids produced in the stomach. In the case of all medications there is no expectation that the underlying cause of the reflux – the weakened diaphragm musculature – will be addressed, merely the severity of the reflux symptoms.

However, in the case of the latter drug class there are significant known side effects. Long-term PPI usage is generally discouraged and several countries insist that clinicians perform a medication review before renewing PPI prescriptions. At least once per year is recommended in the UK [6]. PPI medication is usually not expensive, but the costs of repeat Healthcare Professional (HCP) interventions build to a considerable amount when prescribed for rest-of-life.

PPI drugs belong to one of the safest medication groups, but some research suggests a list of unwanted side effects [7, 8] include increased risk of cardiovascular disease' osteoporosis, dementia, male infertility, diabetes, increased vulnerability to severe covid19 infection.

In addition, harmful bacteria in the stomach like Helicobacter pylori (HP) that would not survive in normal circumstances, can thrive in the weakened acids after PPI treatment. These germs can enter the body and live in the digestive tract. After many years, they can cause sores, called ulcers, in the lining of the stomach or the upper part of the small intestine. For some people, an infection can lead to stomach cancer.

In the UK there are several initiatives in the NHS to reduce PPI prescription, Rotherham [9], All Wales [10] etc.

The final class of treatment is that of surgical intervention. Laparoscopic operations are minimally invasive, whilst other procedures can be more traumatic, all surgical operations carry risks [11]. Such operations require hospitalisation and the National Institute for Health and Care Excellence (NICE) in the UK advise that the cost is GBP 2076 [12].

The prevalence of success of these operations [13] is not 100%. In some cases the remedy is not long lasting and a second operation is required, or the patient will return to PPI medication. Some patients are not deemed suitable for surgery because of other pre-existing factors, and in periods like the Covid19 pandemic such interventions are not prioritised and can be delayed by years.

3. There are several related reflux conditions

Esophagitis is aggravated by acidic reflux and several other conditions are also caused by this condition. All except esophagitis have similar characteristics and treatments.

Reflux is a condition in which stomach acids sometimes bubble up from the stomach, through the oesophagus and into throat, larynx and pharynx. The effect of these acids is to cause the symptoms [14] of:

Heartburn
Burning sensation in the chest
Acidic reflux
Swallowing difficulties
Feeling of a lump in the throat
Feeling of a blockage in the chest when eating
Chest pains
Pain under the breastbone (sternum)
Stomach pains before eating
Stomach pains after eating
Reduced appetite
Early 'Full up' feeling
Feeling sick
Constipated, gassy
Vomiting
Persistent dry or phlegmy cough
Food or drink 'goes down the wrong way'
Hoarseness
Breathing difficulties

It should be noted that if some of the above symptoms are chronic, and especially if they do not respond to medication, they could be caused by cancer or other diseases and these should be considered before diagnosing reflux as the sole cause.

Refluxing stomach acids is the underlying cause of several conditions: LPR, GERD (or GORD), Silent Reflux, IED. These conditions are sometimes known by their full names: Laryngopharyngeal Reflux, Gastroesophageal Reflux Disease, and Intermittent Oesophageal Dysphagia. These various conditions exhibit some or all of the symptoms listed above, they vary slightly but are all caused by the corrosive effect of the refluxed stomach acids. Reflux has an aggravating effect on those with esophagitis.

Another form of reflux is non-acid reflux, this can be diagnosed by impedance and 24-hour pH study. Even though the refluxed stomach contents are not acidic – perhaps due to PPI suppression medication – it is still an unwanted symptom. For this reason, the HH should still be treated even though non-acid reflux is not thought to aggravate esophagitis.

If untreated, the effect of these acids on the oesophagus can lead to inflammation and Barrett's oesophagus. These altered cells can be a sign that they have entered a pre-cancerous phase. It has been shown that even after PPI medication that relieves symptoms, the cancer risk is undiminished [15]. It may be useful to describe the similarities and differences between the various conditions listed.

3.1 GERD

GERD and GORD are the same thing and the name varies only because people spell (o) oesophagus with or without an 'O' in the beginning. It is an abbreviation for Gastroesophageal Reflux Disease.

This condition means that stomach acids bubble up from the stomach, into the oesophagus and up to the throat, larynx and pharynx. The effect of these acids is to cause persistent symptoms like heartburn, a feeling of something stuck in the throat, pain behind the breastbone, difficulties in swallowing some foods, persistent non-productive cough, thick phlegm or frothy saliva, and regurgitation.

3.2 LPR

LPR is an abbreviation for LaryngoPharyngeal Reflux. In this condition stomach acids sometimes bubble up as described earlier and cause the symptoms of heartburn, sore throat, irritation in the larynx and vocal cords, and hoarseness. When the symptoms do not include heartburn, it is often called Silent Reflux instead.

With LPR, unlike similar oesophageal conditions like GERD, the oesophagus itself is not usually irritated, nor does one usually suffer from the impression of something stuck in the throat or behind the breastbone.

3.3 Silent reflux

In this condition stomach acids sometimes bubble up as described earlier and cause the symptoms of sore throat, irritation in the larynx and vocal cords, and hoarseness.

With Silent Reflux, unlike similar oesophageal conditions like GERD, the oesophagus itself is not usually irritated, nor does one usually suffer from the impression of something stuck in the throat or behind the breastbone. Because the symptoms are less obvious than GERD, the condition is known as Silent Reflux. If heartburn is present in addition to the above symptoms the condition is more often described as LPR.

3.4 Heartburn

Heartburn is a condition that everybody experiences occasionally. It is normal after, for example, a heavy meal or fizzy drinks. Constant or persistent heartburn is

SYMPTOM	GERD/GORD	LPR	SILENT REFLUX
Heartburn	●	●	
Lump in the throat	●		
Pain behind the breastbone	●		
Swallowing difficulties	●		
Thick phlegm or frothy saliva	●		
Regurgitation	●		
Persistent cough	●		
Sore throat		●	●
Irritation in the larynx/vocal cords		●	●
Hoarseness		●	●
WHERE?			
Throat	●	●	●
Chest	●		

Figure 1.
Symptom comparisons in reflux diseases.

usually diagnosed by doctors as being caused by reflux which sometimes has the related symptoms of sore throat, irritation in the larynx and vocal cords and hoarseness (**Figure 1**).

4. Hiatus hernia: the root cause of reflux

Reflux of stomach contents can allow the body's own acids to attack the vulnerable soft membranes and tissues in the oesophagus, pharynx, larynx, throat, vocal cords, tongue, and more. Refluxed stomach acids can worsen a pre-existing condition of esophagitis.

The underlying cause of reflux is a muscular weakness in and around the diaphragm where the oesophagus passes through it; this is a Hiatal hernia (HH). Medication will not address this, whereas surgical intervention will, and we will describe later how a new, non-invasive neuromuscular treatment will allow these delinquent muscles to be strengthened and rebuilt as an alternative to surgical intervention.

Many people suffer from reflux but were never diagnosed with HH in earlier internal examinations. The condition is difficult to diagnose with certainty, a sliding HH (90% of all cases) [3, 4] is by its nature intermittent and does not always exhibit at the time of examination. Cuffing of the abdomen to try to provoke herniation is sometimes required to make a diagnosis more certain, especially when using hypopharynx-oesophageal X-ray. It is also the case that the main reason for an internal examination using gastroscopy with biopsy will have been to rule out other serious conditions; not to confirm a HH. Continual pH-monitoring is also used to measure prevalence of acidic reflux but does not aim to identify its cause.

Scientific studies [16–18] have looked at treatment of HH. When recruiting patients to these studies the researchers have always distinguished between those with the symptoms of a HH and a confirmed diagnosis; and those with the symptoms but no confirmation. In these studies, these two groups have the same symptoms, treatment and positive results. In reality there is no difference between the two groups.

In an IQoro customer questionnaire analysis [19] in June 2020 directed at people in Sweden and the UK, self-treating the symptoms of reflux with a neuromuscular device, they were asked how many knew that they had a HH. Most had reflux symptoms and were asked if they had a confirmed diagnosis. More than 2 700 responded: 37% had a confirmation of the condition after examination, and 37% suspected a Hiatal hernia or did not know and had no confirmed diagnosis. In other words, less than 40% of a cohort that probably had a HH had had it confirmed by examination. To add to this uncertainty people were 25% more likely to have had confirmed diagnosis in the UK than in Sweden; suggesting that diagnosis is difficult or not prioritised. Given the paucity of options to treat such a condition it perhaps not surprising that its diagnosis is not deemed important.

4.1 What is hiatus hernia?

Hiatus hernia is not a disease, it is a condition that allows reflux to occur.

The diaphragm is the thin but powerful muscle below the ribcage that divides the chest cavity – where the heart and lungs reside, from the stomach cavity. It is attached to the base of the sternum (breastbone) and follows the base of the ribcage and ends at the spine.

The aperture where the oesophagus passes through the diaphragm is called the Hiatus canal, here the diaphragm muscle grips around the oesophagus and ensures that mouth of the stomach cannot normally intrude upwards into the chest cavity. When the stomach intrudes at other times, in an uncontrolled and undesired way, stomach acids can be refluxed into the oesophagus. During the day, gravity aids the effect of holding the stomach down below the diaphragm, when lying down this effect is not present and is a factor in increased acidic reflux at night.

The valve at the top or mouth of the stomach is called the Lower Oesophageal Sphincter (LES), its job is to remain tightly closed except when swallowing and admitting food and drink into the stomach. An exception to this is when we need to belch, or when we are ill and need to vomit. In these cases, the neck of the stomach slides up through the diaphragm to allow the LES to open upwards to discharge gases or liquids. In its natural position below the diaphragm, it cannot do this. The LES is normally only able to flex open in a downward direction and permit one-way traffic into the stomach. The cause of this uncontrolled intrusion of the neck of the stomach is that the muscle gripping the oesophagus in the Hiatus canal is weakened or ruptured. When held in place below the diaphragm the LES cannot open upwards and allow stomach contents into the oesophagus. The underlying cause of reflux is therefore always a HH.

All babies are born with part of their stomach in the chest cavity; this is normal and usually does not cause a problem. Some, especially those who were born prematurely or in difficult circumstances, may exhibit the symptoms of reflux and projectile vomiting. They may also reject oral feeding; this is due to immaturity of the musculature in the digestive system. At the age of around 6 months the baby's oesophagus starts to grow and lengthen allowing the stomach to descend, and at around 12 months the stomach usually has achieved its correct position below the diaphragm.

5. The weakened diaphragm muscle can be trained like any other

If reflux is allowed by a HH, and this is only a muscle weakness, then why do we treat with medication or by surgical intervention?

If a patient presented with an arm that had atrophied because it had been in a plaster cast for three months, we would not hesitate to recommend a rehab programme based on weights and exercises – and we would not be surprised when it was 100% successful either.

However, there are key differences between the arm muscles and the muscles that need strengthening in the diaphragm.

The arm is made up of skeletally striated muscles that can be commanded by the individual to flex and can therefore be consciously exercised, whereas many of the muscles in the swallowing chain cannot.

Some muscles in the swallowing chain are smooth muscle which are controlled only by the autonomic system - through different command pathways to our voluntary systems.

So, the answer to our question why doctors do not get patients to train this muscle, is that they think that it cannot be done. A patient can be asked to do sit-ups, or lift weights, but not to shut his epiglottis tightly, make peristaltic waves down his oesophagus or squeeze the muscles around his Hiatal canal tightly. Yet it is just this last exercise which is required. The muscles that we need to exercise include these smooth muscles controlled by the body's autonomic system, not only the striated muscles that we can control voluntarily. But we can successfully exercise this musculature back to full strength if we can stimulate the brain stem to issue commands to these muscles. This is the basis of neuromuscular training: the physical exercise stimulates the brain to activate and strengthen the affected smooth muscle.

6. IQoro

IQoro (**Figure 2**) is a simple hand-held neuromuscular treatment device consisting of a curved plastic plate which is inserted pre-dentally by the patient – that is, inside the lips and in front of the teeth. The user grips the handle that protrudes out through his lips, seals his lips and then pulls forward strongly. The partial vacuum thus produced thus triggers the neurological and muscular effects described below. It exercises the muscles in the orofacial and swallowing processes

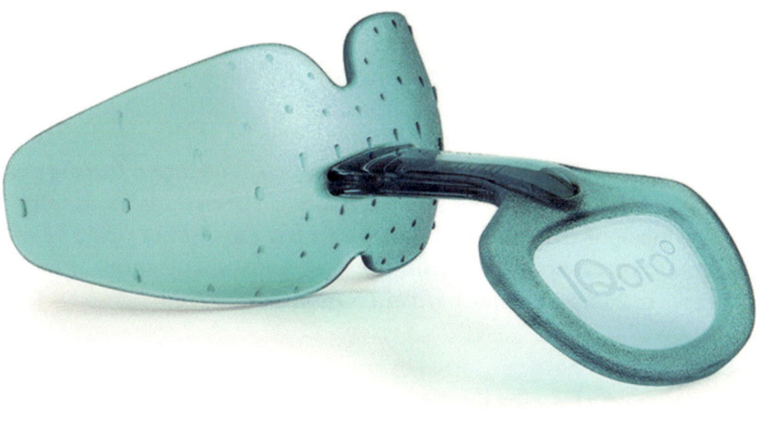

Figure 2.
The IQoro neuromuscular training device.

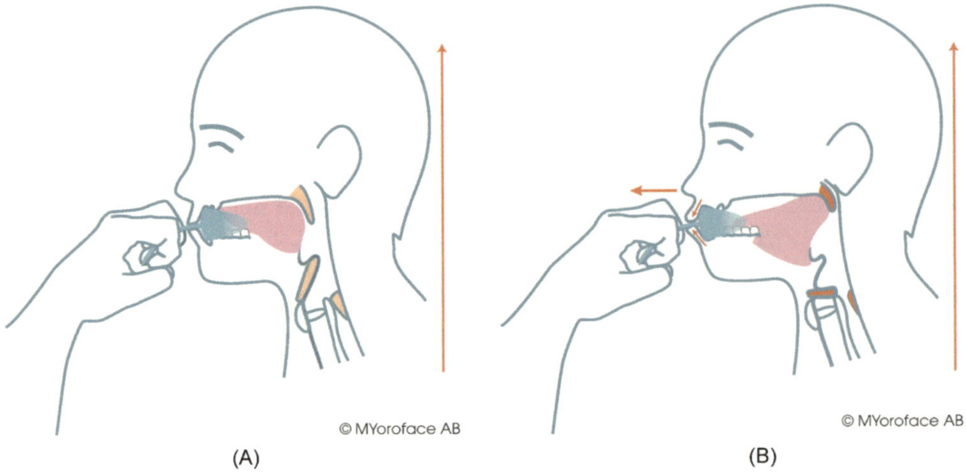

Figure 3.
(A, B). IQoro training regime. (A) the IQoro is inserted pre-dentally, behind closed lips. (B) the patient presses his lips firmly together whilst pulling straight forward strongly for 5–10 seconds, and does this 3 times with 3 seconds rest between each pull. These sessions are performed three times per day, preferably before mealtimes. ***Video 1*** *[20].*

from the face, lips, mouth, throat, airways and oesophagus down to the diaphragm and stomach.

By closing your lips tightly against the handle and pulling the device forward, a low-pressure is created in the oral cavity making the tongue rise and retract and seal against the anterior palatal arch and the soft palate. Further, the naso-pharyngeal and upper airways close, the larynx rises, the epiglottis shuts, and the Upper Oesophageal Sphincter (UES) opens. In other words, the exercise action provokes the mechanical components of a swallow. The UES is also known as the Posterior Oesophageal Sphincter (PES).

These physical movements alone are not enough to strengthen the weakened musculature in the diaphragm; indeed the muscles that need to be targeted to repair the hernia lie around and outside the oesophagus. No amount of low pressure flexing the oesophagus can have a direct effect on the muscles in the hiatal canal around the oesophagus.

Instead, they are exercised by proxy, the muscle and organ movements described above promote intense stimuli in the afferent Cranial Nerves to the brainstem. Here they provoke a sensory motoric reflex arc that causes messages to be issued through the efferent, motor nerves to the muscles in the swallowing chain. Crucially, this includes the smooth musculature that can only be commanded by the autonomic system.

In this way, for example, the long outer muscles that run down along the side of the oesophagus and fasten below the diaphragm, by the hiatal canal, are activated. As they flex, they pull on the weakened musculature around the hiatal canal and this musculature is exercised and strengthened.

The training regime (**Figure 3** A, B; Video 1) was developed during research studies; optimal training is three such pulls, each of 10 seconds' duration, and repeated three times per day, totally 90 seconds per day. Some positive effect on reflux symptoms is often noticed within the first month, and more than 60% of respondents reported improvement within 5 months [19, 20].

7. The neurology of the swallowing process

Understanding the neurology a little more deeply is therefore key for those who wish to understand neuromuscular training more fully.

The process of transmitting food and drink into the stomach is called the swallowing process, this also includes the process by which food and drink are held in the stomach and not refluxed. Hence a HH disrupts a normal swallowing process.

When food is to be eaten it is first processed using the voluntary muscles in the jaw, lips and tongue. As the bolus is pushed back to the pharynx by the action of the tongue base rising and retracting, the voluntary part of the process ends; the rest is reflexive.

Four sensory Cranial Nerves (*CN*) are primarily involved in the swallowing process. Stimulation of the *CN (V) Trigeminus* in the lips is the first step. In short order thereafter, the *CN (IX) Glossopharyngeus* and *CN (X) Vagus* nerves are also triggered, and then in turn the *CN (V) Trigeminus and CN (VII) Facialis* nerve too in the soft palate and anterior palate (**Figure 4**).

In the brain stem we find the *Nucleus Tractus Solitarius* (NTS), the afferent nucleus. The NTS is the core that gathers all incoming sensory signals from the lips, oral cavity and pharynx via the afferent nerve pathways, and transmits them either to the brain's cortex or directly to the network-like system in the brain stem called the *Formatio Reticularis* (FR). The FR not only controls the swallowing process, but also the respiratory and swallowing processes, cough reflex, orofacial and postural control, vomiting, bowel and bladder evacuation, these are all indivisibly interlinked at the neurological level, where the *Formatio Reticularis* plays a central role in governing all the muscles involved in these functions.

The three swallowing centres in the brain stem are triggered in the following sequence. The first swallowing centre interprets that something is to be swallowed, and this instruction is sent to the second swallowing centre.

The second swallowing centre transmits signals to the muscles via the motor nerves – the downward-transmitting efferent nerve pathways. Here, there is a pre-programmed 'go/no-go' decision: 'swallow' or 'do not swallow' - a so-called stereotypical muscle response. When something is to be swallowed the command is first sent to the *Nucleus Ambiguus* (NA) an efferent nucleus which, in its turn, sends the instruction to swallow to the major components of the swallowing musculature via the motor, efferent nerve pathways to the skeletally striated muscles. Concurrently, impulses are also sent to the third swallowing centre.

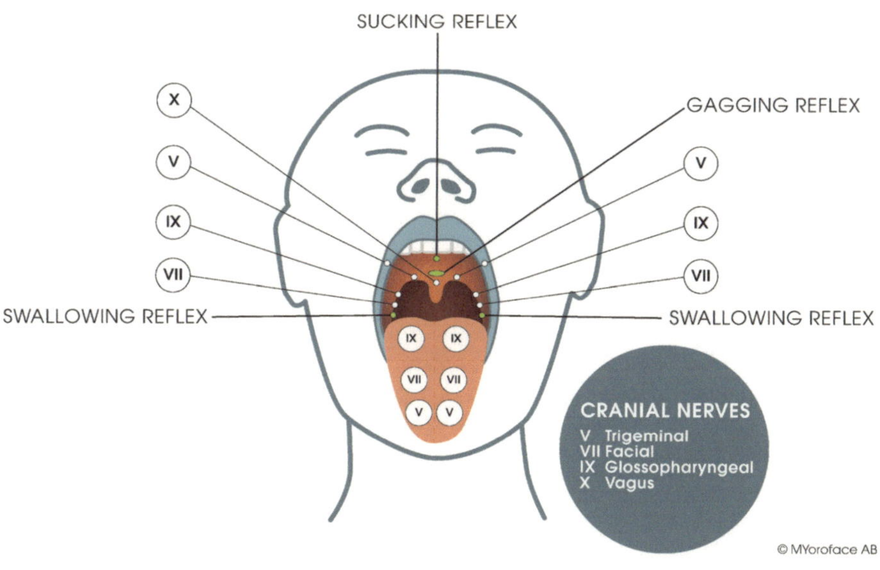

Figure 4.
Cranial nerves and reflex points in the oral cavity.

The five motor nerves that are important for swallowing are: *CN Trigeminus (V)*, *CN Facialis (VII)*, *CN Glossopharyngeus (IX)*, *CN Vagus (X)* and *CN Hypoglossus (XII)*. The first four are both sensory (afferent) and motor (efferent) nerve pathways.

The third swallowing centre transmits information to the *Nucleus Dorsalis Nervi Vagi* (NDNV) an efferent nucleus, and then onwards to the smooth muscles including those in the oesophagus (**Figures** 5 and **6**).

The three swallowing centres' interactions - from brain stem to muscles.

These signals are transmitted via efferent nerves that can be thought of as cables containing various fibres, motor neurons, to the muscles and glands. There are three different kinds of motor neurons that are important in the swallowing process.

- The *General Somatic Efferent* (GSE) motor neurones are present in the *CN Hypoglossus (XII)* and *CN Oculomotorius (III)* which transmit signals onwards to the tongue's and the inner eyes' voluntary skeletal striated muscles musculature.

- The *Special Visceral Efferent (SVE)* motor neurons act through the *CN Trigeminus (V)*, *CN Facialis (VII)*, *CN Glossopharyngeus (IX)*, *CN Vagus (X)* and *CN Accessorius (XI)* which transmit signals to the voluntary musculature in

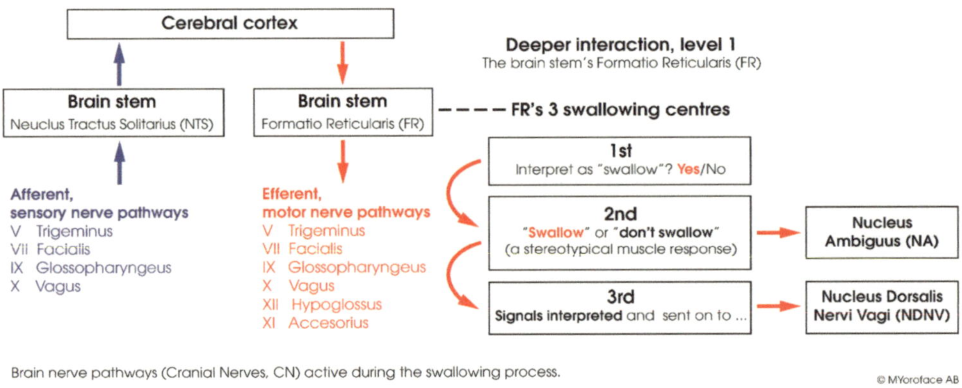

Figure 5.
The sensory-motor reflex arc (level 1). The three swallowing centres' interactions - from brain stem to muscles.

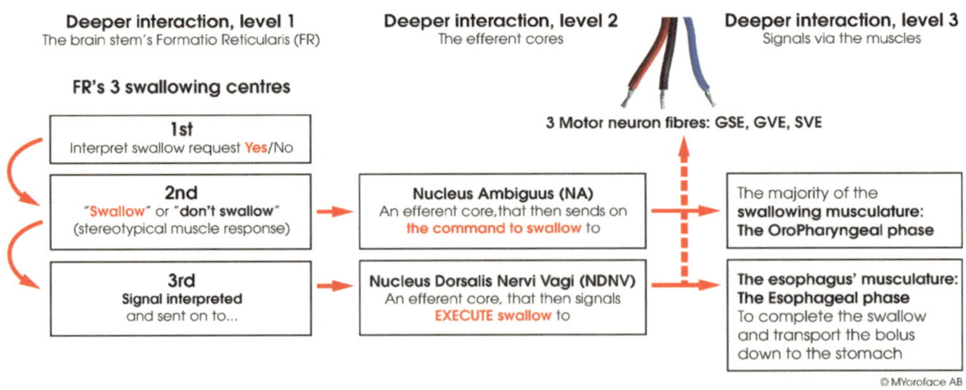

Figure 6.
The sensory-motor reflex arc (level 1–3). The three swallowing centres′ interactions from: - the 2nd Centre to the striated muscles - the 3rd Centre to the smooth muscles.

the mouth, chewing muscles, facial musculature, pharynx, larynx, oesophagus and diaphragm.

- The *General Visceral Efferent (GVE)* motor neurons act via *CN Facialis (VII)* and *CN Glossopharyngeus (IX)* which transmit signals to the glands, blood vessels and smooth muscles in the pharynx, stomach and rectum.

The signal pathways from the above-named motor neurons are:
CN (V) Trigeminus – signals via the SVE.
CN (VII) Facialis – signals via the SVE and the GVE.
CN (IX) Glossopharyngeus – signals via the SVE and GVE.
CN (X) Vagus – signals via the SVE.
CN (XII) Hypoglossus – signals via the GSE.

The sum of all the above signals initiates a pre-programmed cooperation between the 148 muscles that are involved in the transport of each food bite from the mouth down to the stomach. Controlled by these circuits and executed by these muscles. Breathing and postural control function are stimulated and strengthened, as are the tongue, soft palate and When using IQoro as a neuromuscular training device it triggers the sensory-motor reflex arc described earlier. This manifests itself in improvement in swallowing including the weakened diaphragm muscles that allow reflux, and then successively in other functions pharynx (**Figure** 7).

So, we have two effects of IQoro on the muscles. One is both neurological and physiological (the upper muscle chain from the lips to the upper part of the oesophagus) promoting movement, flexion and strengthening; and a second one, with only a neurological effect (the lower part of the oesophagus to the rectum).

The efferent nerves send signals to the muscles and glands through the following motor neurons:

Motor neuron fibres	Cranial nerves	Muscles and glands
General Somatic Efferent (GSE) 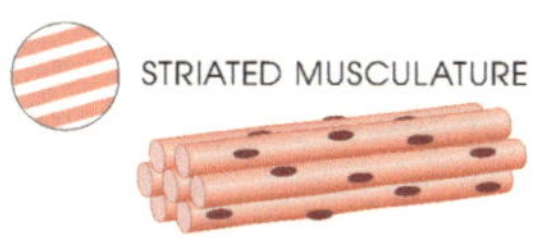 STRIATED MUSCULATURE	XII Hypoglossus III Oculomotorius	Tongue Eyes' inner muscles
Special Visceral Efferent (SVE) 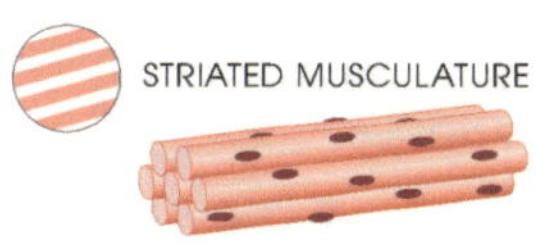 STRIATED MUSCULATURE	V Trigeminus m. tensor tympani VII Facialis m. stapedius IX Glossopharyngeus X Vagus XI Accessorius	Face Oral cavity Chewing muscles Eyes' outer muscles Pharynx Larynx Esophagus Diaphragm
General Visceral Efferent (GVE) 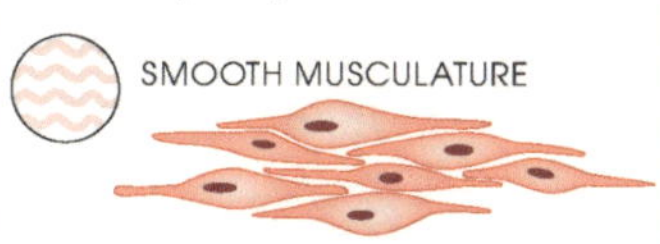 SMOOTH MUSCULATURE	VII Facialis IX Glossopharyngeus	Glands Blood vessels Smooth musculature

Figure 7.
The three motor neuron fibres, their nerves and effect organ connections.

8. Scientific evidence of the effectiveness of neuromuscular treatment

The effectiveness of neuromuscular training is supported by more than a dozen scientific studies conducted at university hospitals in Sweden. This section will present abstracts from three studies that are of particular relevance to HH and reflux.

In all three studies [16–18] quoted here the patients were long-term users of PPI medication before the studies began. In a Medtech Innovation Briefing [21] produced by the UK's National Institute for Health and Care Excellence in 2019 they quoted, "all patients continued with their PPI medication as advised. As symptoms reduced, patients ceased to medicate. Use or cessation of PPIs was under the control of the patients' doctors. At end-of-training in the 3 studies quoted 93%, 58% and 61% that they ceased all PPI medication, the remainder mostly reduced dose and intake frequency". For this reason, medication can be excluded as the cause for improvement.

Overall, the studies showed success rates in the region of 98%, this is the same result reported by IQoro customers [19] in a survey conducted in 2020.

In these scientific studies of neuromuscular training there was particular focus on measurement methods. Patients were recruited as suffering from intermittent oesophageal dysphagia (IED) and reflux despite PPI medication from 1 year to many years and this was confirmed by a comprehensive test battery.

The test methodologies used were:

- Symptom Questionnaire [14].
- Visual Analogue Scale (VAS) [22] in which the patient records the ability to swallow food.
- Orofacial Motor Tests (OFMT) [23] and Orofacial Sensory Tests (OFST) [24] were carried out in order to exclude patients whose dysphagia were of central nervous origin. All tests showed normal brain function.
- Pharyngeal Sling Force (PSF) [25], measuring the resistance of the buccinator mechanism,
- Velopharyngeal Closure Test (VCT) [26] testing velum closure competence.
- Timed Water Swallow Test (TWST) [27] measuring swallowing competence and aspiration.
- PSF, VCT and TWST were used to confirm both normal oropharyngeal function and training compliance.
- High Resolution Manometry (HRM) [28] measuring pressure changes in the UES and the diaphragmatic hiatus.

In all cases tests were made in the recruiting process, at baseline, and at end-of-treatment; however, all patients were contacted by telephone or in the clinic two or three times to verify compliance before follow-up at end-of-treatment.

8.1 Oesophageal dysphagia and reflux symptoms before and after oral

IQoro® training. Hägg M, Tibbling L, Franzén T.
World J Gastroenterol 2015; 21(24): 7558–7562.
DOI: 10.3748 / wjg.v21.i24.7558 [16].

Study type

Peer reviewed, Prospective, Cohort pre- and post- study.

Aim

To examine whether training with an IQoro Neuromuscular Training (IQNT) improves oesophageal dysphagia and reflux symptoms.

Patients

43 patients (F = 22, M = 21) median age 57 years (range 22–85) with oesophageal dysphagia of a non-stenotic nature for a median period of 3 years (range: 1–15 years), of which:

- 21 patients with median age 52 years (range 19–85) with a confirmed Hiatal hernia,
- 22 patients with median age 57 years (range 22–85) exhibited Hiatal hernia symptoms but had no confirmed diagnosis.

All patients had been using PPI medication for more than one year.

Methods

IQoro training (**Figure 3** A, B; Video 1), 3 x 10 seconds three times a day, totally 90 seconds per day, for a duration of 6 months. Outcome measurements were made at two time points: before training and at end of training.

Outcome measurements

Patients (n = 12), median age 53 years (range 22–68 years) with hiatal hernia were measured using:

- High Resolution Manometry during IQoro traction to record pressure in [28]:
  - the UES (normal restin pressure > 30 mmHg, **Table 1**).
  - the diaphragmatic pressure in the hiatus canal (normal resting pressure 10–35 mm HG, **Table 1**).

All patients were measured using:

- Symptom questionnaire (IED = intermittent oesophageal dysphagia a sensation of solid food retention in the chest at swallowing, acid chest symptoms and/or acid regurgitation), scored 0–3: 0 = no, 1 = slight, 2 = moderate, 3 = severe [14].
- Swallowing questionnaire (ability to swallow food), measured using
  - Visual Analogue Scale (VAS 0–100: 0 = normal, 100 = total inability) [22],.

Items	UES n = 12	Hiatus n = 12
Resting pressure	68 (40–110)	0 (0–0)
IQS traction	95 (80–130)	65 (20–100)

Data are mean (range) mmHg.

Table 1.
Oesophageal high resolution manometry pressures in the upper oesophageal sphincter (UES) and hiatus during rest and traction with an oral IQoro screen (IQS) in patients with hiatal hernia.

- Pharyngeal sling force (measured using Lip Force meter) [25],.
    - o lower normal value ≥15 N
- Velopharyngeal Closure Test (VCT) [26],.
    - o lower normal value ≥10 sec
- Orofacial motor tests [23],.
- Orofacial sensory tests (oral stereognosia and two-point discrimination) [24].

Results

All Orofacial motor tests and Orofacial sensory test scores were normal before treatment, indicating that there was no neurological cause to the patient's symptoms.

No significant difference in symptom frequency was found between the group with confirmed hiatus hernia, and those without a confirmed diagnosis, this was true both before and after training.

- Oesophageal dysphagia was present in all 43 patients at start of treatment, and 98% of patients showed improvement after IQoro neuromuscular training ($p < 0.001$).
- Reflux symptoms were reported before training in 86% of the patients, 100% of these showed improvement at end of training, ($p < 0.001$) and 58% were entirely symptom free and ceased PPI medication.
- VAS scores were classified as pathologic in all 43 patients, and 100% showed improvement after IQoro neuromuscular training ($p < 0.001$).
- Pharyngeal sling force test values ($p < 0.001$) were significantly higher after IQoro neuromuscular training.
- Velopharyngeal closure test values ($p < 0.001$) were significantly higher after IQoro neuromuscular training.
- High Resolution Manometry during IQoro traction showed an increase in mean pressure in the diaphragmatic hiatus region from 0 mm Hg at rest (range: 0–0 mm Hg) to 65 mm Hg (range: 20–100 mm Hg, **Table 1**).

Statistical significance of result

($p < 0.001$) oesophageal dysphagia.
($p < 0.001$) reflux symptoms.
($p < 0.001$) VAS values.
($p < 0.001$) pharyngeal sling force scores significantly higher.
($p < 0.001$) VCT scores significantly higher.
(p = NS) No statistical difference between symptoms or outcomes between those with or without confirmed Hiatal hernia diagnosis - both before and after treatment.

Conclusion

IQoro neuromuscular training can relieve/improve oesophageal dysphagia and reflux symptoms in adults, likely due to improved hiatal competence. The similarity of the results in the two groups suggest that many people suffer from Hiatus hernia despite this not having been confirmed by diagnosis.

8.2 Effect of IQoro® training in hiatal hernia patients with misdirected

swallowing and oesophageal retention symptoms. Hägg M, Tibbling L, **Franzén T. Acta Otolaryngol. 2015 Jul;135 (7):635–639.**
DOI: 10.3109/00016489.2015.1016185 [17].

Study type

Peer reviewed, Prospective, Cohort pre- and post-study.

Aim

To investigate whether muscle training with IQoro influences symptoms of misdirected swallowing and oesophageal retention in patients with hiatal hernia.

Patients

28 patients, F = 14, M = 14. Adult, Median age 59 years (range 22–85). All patients had hiatal hernia with misdirected swallowing and oesophageal retention symptoms for median 4 years (range 1–28).

Methods

IQoro training (**Figure 3** A, B; Video 1) of duration 3 x 10 seconds three times per day for a duration of 6–8 months. Outcome measurements were made at two time points: before and at end of training.

Outcome measurements

12 patients in the study

- High Resolution Manometry (HRM) [28].

All patients in the study,

- Symptom Questionnaire typical for HH [14],.
- Visual Analogue Scale – VAS – self assessed scoring [22],.
- Pharyngeal sling force (using Lip Force meter) [25],.
    - lower normal value ≥15 N,
- Velopharyngeal Closure Test (VCT) [26],.
    - lower normal value ≥10 sec
- Swallowing ability (measured using Timed Water Swallow Test - TWST) [27],.
    - lower normal value for swallowing rate ≥ 10 ml / sec
- Orofacial Motor Test [23],.
- Orofacial Sensory Test (oral stereognosia and two-point discrimination) [24],.

Results

All Orofacial motor tests and Orofacial sensory test scores were normal before treatment, indicating that there was no neurological cause to the patient's symptoms.

- Reflux symptoms were reported before training in 100% of patients, 100% of these showed improvement at end of training, ($p < 0.001$) and 61% were entirely symptom free and ceased PPI medication.
- All hiatal hernia patients were improved after training ($p < 0.001$) with IQoro and showed significant improvements in
    - o misdirected swallowing
    - o cough,
    - o hoarseness,
    - o oesophageal retention
    - o globus sensation,
    - o VAS, Pharyngeal Sling Force (PSF = LFT), VCT and TWST = SCT.
- Traction during the training action with IQoro resulted in a 65 mm Hg increase in the mean pressure of the Diaphragmatic Hiatus as measured by high resolution manometry (**Table 1**).

Statistical significance of result

($p < 0.001$) improvements in misdirected swallowing, cough, hoarseness, oesophageal retention, globus sensation, VAS scores, pharyngeal sling force, velopharyngeal closure and swallowing ability.

Conclusion

IQoro training significantly improves all the symptoms of hiatus hernia, potentially through improved hiatal competence. All symptoms were significantly improved at end of training suggesting that lasting improved hiatal competence had been achieved.

8.3 Oral neuromuscular training relieves hernia-related dysphagia and GERD symptoms as effectively in obese as in non-obese patients.

Franzén T., Tibbling L., Hägg M. Acta Oto-Laryngol.
Jan 2019;138 (11):1–5 DOI: 0.1080/00016489.2018.1503715 [18].

Study type

Peer reviewed, Prospective, Clinical Study, Cohort pre- and post- study.

Aim

To investigate whether Body Mass Index (BMI) has significance on IQoro neuromuscular training's effectiveness in treating Hiatal hernia (HH) related symptoms.

Patients

86 adult patients (F = 46, M = 40) with verified HH and long- standing Intermittent Oesophageal Disease (IED) and other Gastro Oesophageal Reflux Disease (GERD) symptoms.

Before entry into the study the patients were partitioned into three groups according to BMI (**Table 2**):

- Group A:
    - o normal weight, BMI < 25

- (n = 37: 19 women of median age 68 yrs., 18 men, median 72 yrs.)
- GERD symptoms - median duration 5 yrs. (1–75).
- PPI medication history median 5 yrs.

- Group B:
    - moderately obese, BMI 25–29
    - (n = 28: 16 women of median age 59 yrs., 12 men of median age 56 yrs.)
    - GERD symptoms - median duration 6 yrs. (1–15).
    - PPI medication history median 6 yrs.
- Group C:
    - severely obese, BMI 30–37
    - (n = 21: 11 women of median age 52 yrs., 10 men of median age 70 yrs.
    - GERD symptoms - median duration 3 yrs. (1–29).
    - PPI medication history median 3 yrs.

Methods

All patients received IQoro neuromuscular training 3 x 10 seconds, three times per day for a duration of 6 months.

All patients were measured before and after treatment.

Outcome measurements

Radiology or gastroscopy was used to confirm HH and to rule out oesophageal stenosis before inclusion.

An Orofacial Motor Test (OFMT) and an Orofacial Sensory Test (OST) were performed in order to exclude symptoms of any central nervous lesion. Patients with neurological diseases were excluded.

All patients were measured before and after treatment using:

- Symptom questionnaire regarding IED and GERD (reflux, heartburn, chest pain, dysphagia, globus sensation, non-productive cough, hoarseness, and misdirected swallowing) [14]

Items	Group A; *n* = 37	Group B; *n* = 28	Group C; *n* = 21
Median age	69 yrs. (20–85)	57 yrs. (22–85)	62 yrs. (44–87)
Gender	19 women, 18 men	16 women, 12 men	11 women, 10 men
GERD symptom duration	5 yrs. (1–75)	6 yrs. (1–15)	3 yrs. (1–29)
BMI before/after IQNT	23 (17–24) / 23 (20–25)	28 (26–29) / 27 (24–29)	33 (30–37) / 31 (27–38)

Ranges in parentheses. BMI and GERD: median values; IQNT: Neuromuscular training with an oral IQoro.

Table 2.
Age, gender, symptom duration, and BMI in groups a, B, and C.

- Swallowing ability (measured using Timed Water Swallow Test - TWST) [27]
  - lower normal value for swallowing rate ≥ 10 ml/sec
- Pharyngeal sling force (measured using Lip Force meter) [25]
  - lower normal value ≥15 N
- Swallowing questionnaire (ability to swallow food) [22]
  - measured using Visual Analogue Scale (VAS 0–100)

Results

- At entry into the study there were no significant differences between the three BMI groups in:
  - TWST = SCT, PSF = LFT or VAS values
  - IED and GERD symptom severity, except that:
    a. heartburn and cough were significantly more common in Groups B (moderately obese) and C (severely obese), and that
    b. misdirected swallowing was significantly more common in Group C (severely obese).
- After **IQoro** neuromuscular training the following was observed in all three BMI groups:
  - all IED and GERD symptom scores were significantly improved or reduced ($p < 0.001$).
  - median BMI was not significantly changed.
  - self-assessed GERD symptom improvement showed no significant difference across the groups, except for heartburn, cough and misdirected swallowing which were significantly ($p < 0.01$) more reduced in obese patients than in normal bodyweight patients.
  - TWST = SCT and pharyngeal sling force (LFT) and VAS score, showed significant improvement ($p < 0.001$) in median values, with no significant difference between the BMI groups except for:
    a. TWST values, which were significantly ($p < 0.01$) more improved in Group C (severely obese) than in Group A (normal weight).
    b. pharyngeal sling force (LFT), which was significantly ($p < 0.05$) more improved in Group B (moderately obese) than in Group A (normal weight).

Statistical significance of result

($p < 0.001$) all IED and GERD symptom scores were significantly improved or reduced.

($p < 0.01$) heartburn, cough and misdirected swallowing were significantly more reduced in obese patients than in normal bodyweight patients.

($p < 0.001$) VAS score, TWST, and pharyngeal sling force (LFT) improved.

($p <$ NS) no significant difference between other results across the three groups.

Conclusion

IQoro neuromuscular training (IQNT), a non-surgical treatment for IED and other GERD symptoms in hiatal hernia patients, is equally successful in treating moderately- or severely obese patients as in treating sufferers of normal weight. Obesity in itself does not therefore seem to be a handicap in treating IED and other GERD symptoms by IQNT.

9. Importance of neuromuscular treatment

Orally administered neuromuscular treatment as described, deserves wider deployment and, where more evidence is deemed necessary, further research. Unlike medication it treats the root cause of reflux, and without the cost and inconvenience of surgical intervention. It is self-administered by the patient and instructions for use are clearly explained in the accompanying manual; in surveys 98% thought that instructions were clear, and 97% thought it was easy to start training [19]. PPI drugs should not be re-prescribed routinely but rather only after a medication review; these reviews are often planned twice per year and add a burden to primary care practices. The drugs themselves have a considerable cost over the course of a patient's lifetime. An IQoro sells singly at around €150.

The overall advantage is that it addresses and treats the underlying condition, not merely the symptoms.

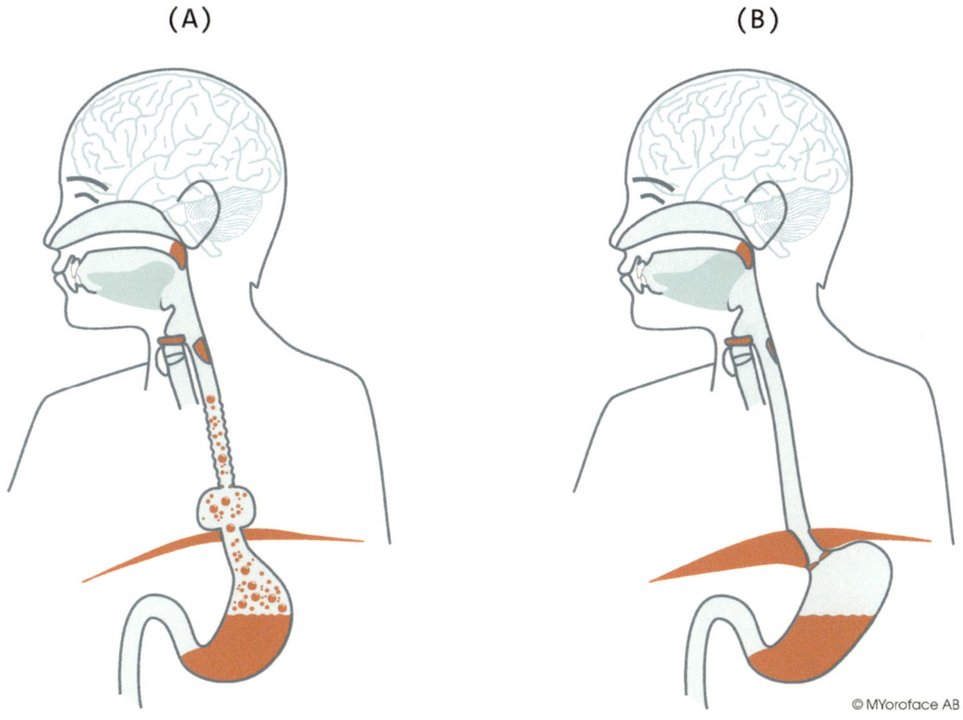

Figure 8.
(A) Sliding hiatal hernia; (B) functional anatomy (A) ***sliding hiatal hernia.*** *The upper part of the stomach has slid up through the hiatal canal. This causes difficulties with opening the PES and allows gastroesophageal reflux. (B)* ***Normal anatomy.*** *The neck of the stomach is correctly held below the diaphragm promoting normal PES function and preventing reflux.*

10. Conclusions

Esophagitis is a debilitating condition that is made worse by the effects of refluxed stomach acids. Reflux is caused by a Hiatus hernia, a weakening in the diaphragm muscles where the oesophagus passes through to join to the stomach (**Figure 8**). These weakened muscles can be compensated for by surgical intervention, or the amount and strength of the stomach acids produced can by reduced by medication. The most commonly prescribed drugs are Proton Pump Inhibitors, these carry proven unwanted side-effects.

Neuromuscular exercise is a safe, natural and simple treatment that can be carried out by the patient his or herself, and the underlying cause of the reflux is proven to be treated in 97% [16–18] of cases.

Acknowledgements

The authors would like to thank Terry Morris for his assistance in authoring this chapter, for creating the summary of abstracts from which the three studies above are copied, and performing the data analysis on the '2020 Vision' customer survey referred to above. The studies reproduced above were supported by grants from The Centre for Research & Development, Uppsala University/County Council of Gävleborg, Gävle, Sweden, and The Council for Regional Research in Uppsala and Örebro region, Sweden.

Conflict of interest

IQoro® is patented and CE-marked by MYoroface AB. Mary Hägg is the inventor.

Swedish patent SE 1350314–9, 2014 July 14. IQoro is a Class 1 Medical Device for therapeutic use. The authors, Mary Hägg and Thomas Franzén declare that they have no conflict of interest.

Notes/thanks/other declarations

The study was performed according to the Helsinki Declaration. Informed written and verbal consent was obtained from all the participants in the studies. All images are kindly provided by MYoroface AB.

Author details

Mary Hägg[1,2]* and Thomas Franzén[3]*

1 Department of Otorhinolaryngology, Speech and Swallowing Centre, Hudiksvall Hospital, Sweden

2 Centre for Research and Development, Uppsala University/Region Gävleborg, Sweden

3 Department of Surgery and Department of Clinical and Experimental Medicine, Linköping University, Norrköping, Sweden

*Address all correspondence to: mary.hagg@regiongavleborg.se; mary@myoroface.com; thomas.franzen@regionostergotland.se

References

[1] Choueiri NE, Prather CM. Choueiri NE, et al. Barrett's esophagus: a pre-cancerous condition approach to diag nosis and management. Mo Med. 2009 Sep-Oct;106(5):339–42. PMID: 19902713

[2] Yu HX, Han CS, Xue JR, et al. Esophageal hiatal hernia: risk, diagnosis and management. Expert Rev Gastroenterol Hepatol. 2018;12(4):319–29.

[3] Siegal SR, Dolan JP, Hunter JG. Modern diagnosis and treatment of hiatal hernias. Langenbecks Arch Surg. 2017;402(8):1145–51.

[4] Johansson KE, Ask P, Boeryd B, Fransson SG, Tibbling L. Oesophagitis, signs of reflux, and gastric acid secretion in patients with symptoms of gastro-oesophageal reflux disease. Scand J Gastroenterol 1986;21:837–847 [PMID: 3775250]

[5] Stein E, Sloan J, Sonu I, et al. GERD for the nongastroenterologist: successful evaluation, management, and lifestyle-based symptom control. Ann N Y Acad Sci. 2020 Dec;1482(1):106–112. DOI: 10.1111/nyas.14496.

[6] National Institute for Health and Care Excellence. Gastro-oesophageal reflux disease and dyspepsia in adults: investigation and management. (September 2014) (CG184). Available at: www.nice.org.uk/guidance/cg184/resources/gastrooesophageal-ref lux-disease-and-dyspepsia-inadults-investigation-and-management-35109812699845

[7] Bjornsson E, Abrahamsson H, Simren M et al. Discontinuation of proton pump inhibitors in patients on long-term therapy: A double-blind, placebo-controlled trial. Ailment Pharmacol Ther. 2006; 24(6): 945–954

[8] Saman Chubineh, John Birk. Proton pump inhibitors: the good, the bad, and the unwanted. South Med J. 2012 Nov; 105(11):613–618. DOI: 10.1097/SMJ.0b013e31826efbea.

[9] NHS, Rotherham, Clinical Commissioning Group, Guidance to Review Proton Pump Inhibitors (PPIs) prescribing, Eloise Summerfield May 2019

[10] All Wales Therapeutics and Toxicology Centre. All Wales Proton Pump Inhibitor and dyspepsia resource pack. Material to support appropriate prescribing of Proton Pump Inhibitors across Wales. April 2013 http://www.awmsg.org/docs/awmsg/medman/All%20Wales%20Proton%20Pump%20Inhibitor%20and%20Dyspepsia%20Resource%20Pack.pdf

[11] Maret-Ouda J, Wahlin K, Artama M, et al. Risk of Esophageal Adenocarcinoma After Antireflux Surgery in Patients With Gastroesophageal Reflux Disease in the Nordic Countries. JAMA Oncol. Published online August 23, 2018. DOI: 10.1001/jamaoncol.2018.3054

[12] Costing statement: Dyspepsia and gastro-oesophageal reflux disease. https://www.nice.org.uk/guidance/cg184/resources/costing-statement-pdf-193164877

[13] D Mayo, A Darbyshire, S Mercer, et al. Technique and outcome of day case laparoscopic hiatus hernia surgery for small and large hernias: a five-year retrospective reflux as a risk factor for esophageal adenocarcinoma. N Engl J Med. 1999;340(11):825–31.review from a high-volume UK centre. Ann R Coll Surg Engl. 2020 Oct;102(8):611–615. DOI: 10.1308/rcsann.2020.0151. Epub 2020 Jul 31.

[14] Franzén T, Boström J, Tibbling Grahn L, et al. Prospective study of symptoms and gastro-oesophageal reflux 10 years after posterior partial fundoplication. Br J Surg. 1999;86:956–

960. DOI: 10.1046/j.1365-2168.1999.01183.x.

[15] Lagergren J, Bergstrom R, Lindgren A, Nyren O. Symptomatic gastroesophageal reflux as a risk factor for esophageal adenocarcinoma. N Engl J Med. 1999;340(11):825–831.

[16] Hägg M, Tibbling L, Franzén T. Esophageal dysphagia and reflux symptoms before and after oral IQoro® training. World J Gastroenterol 2015;21 (24):7558–7562. Open access: http://www.wjgnet.com/1007-9327/full/v21/i24/7558.htm

[17] Hägg M, Tibbling L, Franzén T. Effect of IQoro® training in hiatal hernia patients with misdirected swallowing and esophageal retention symptoms. Acta Otolaryngol. 2015;135 (7):635–639.

[18] Franzén T., Tibbling L., Hägg M. Oral neuromuscular training relieves hernia- related dysphagia and GERD symptoms as effectively in obese as in non-obese patients. Acta Otolaryngol. 2018 Nov;138(11):1004–1008. DOI: 10.1080/00016489.2018.1503715. Epub 2019 Jan 10.

[19] PPT 1_Cust survey 2020 IQoro MYoroface, June 2020.

[20] Video 1_IQoro_This is how you exercise_EN_short version

[21] Medtech Innovation Briefing produced by the UK's National Institute for Health and Care Excellence in 2019. Available from: https://www.nice.org.uk/advice/mib176

[22] Joyce CR, Zutshi DW, Hrubes VF, et al. Comparison of fixed interval and visual analogue scales for rating chronic pain. Eur J Clin Pharmacol. 1975;8:415–420.

[23] Hägg M, Larsson B. Effects of motor and sensory stimulation in stroke patients with long-lasting dysphagia. Dysphagia 2004; 19:219–230 [PMID: 15667056]

[24] Calhoun KH, Gibson B, Hartley L, Minton J, Hokanson JA. Age-related changes in oral sensation. Laryngoscope 1992; 102:109–116 [PMID: 1738279]

[25] Hägg M, Olgarsson M, Anniko M. Reliable lip force measurement in healthy controls and in patients with stroke: a methodologic study. Dysphagia 2008; 23: 291–296 [PMID: 18253790 DOI: 10.1007/s00455-007-9143-y]

[26] Netsell R, Hixon TJ. A noninvasive method for clinically estimating subglottal air pressure. J Speech Hear Disord 1978; 43: 326–330 [PMID: 692098]

[27] Nathadwarawala KM, Nicklin J, Wiles CM. A timed test of swallowing capacity for neurological patients. J Neurol Neurosurg Psychiatry 1992;55: 822–5.

[28] Tibbling L, Gezelius P, Franzén T. Factors influencing lower esophageal sphincter relaxation after deglutition. World J Gastroenterol 2011; 17: 2844–2847 [PMID: 21734792 DOI: 10.3748/wjg. v17.i23.2844]

Section 3

Gastritis

Chapter 6

Pathophysiology of *H. pylori*

Karam Dawood and Israa Mamdooh

Abstract

Helicobacter species were known for long as a causative agent of gastritis. *H. pylori* associated gastritis is characterized by the presence of acute and chronic inflammation. Previously, it was believed that in *H. pylori* gastritis, fundic inflammation was less important than that of the antral mucosa. However, *H. pylori* and gastroesophageal reflux disease create, or arise concurrently, may also be caused by the anatomical role of the inflammatory cell infiltrate. The source of *H. pylori* is mostly unknown. *H. pylori* has a small host range and is present in people and some non-human primates nearly exclusively. In rare cases, the presence of pets may be a concern for *H. pylori* infection; hence, pets should be isolated. There is also no definitive proof for zoonotic *H. pylori* transmission. The direct transmission from person to person, either oral or fecal-oral route or both, is expected to lead to new infections. *H. pylori* colonization is not an infection itself, but it impacts the relative likelihood that multiple pathological conditions of the upper gastrointestinal tract and even the hepatobiliary tract will grow. Therefore, *H. pylori* examination alone is not relevant but can be done in order to ascertain the cause of a basic disorder, such as peptic ulcer disease or to avoid disease, for example in subjects with family gastric carcinoma. A positive test result will validate the procedure, and a negative test result can suggest that other etiological causes or prevention steps needs to be examined. Gastritis is divided into acute and chronic. Several virulence factors play a role in the disease such as *cag* PAI (Pathogenicity Island) and VacA vacuolating cytotoxin. Different adhesins and their receptors aid in *H. pylori* colonization and invasion. Based on analogy with other mucosal infections, it was initially assumed that a protective immune response against *H. pylori* would predominantly be mediated by antibodies. Subsequent experiments have indicated that the relevance of the humoral system for protective immunity is only marginal. Antibodies can effectively prevent infection and reduce colonization in animal models.

Keywords: Helicobacter, Gastritis, CAG pathogenicity island, Vac A vaculating cytotoxin, Autoantibodies

1. Introduction

1.1 History of gastritis

Warren and Marshall in 1983 first recorded *H. pylori's* relationship of gastric mucosa in adults with antral gastritis [1]. Shortly thereafter, Hill *et al.*, four children who were afflicted with *H. pylori* had identified chronic mononuclear cell gastritis [2]. That same year, Cadranel and colleagues described organisms present in eight children with chronic, lymphocytic gastritis [3]. Subsequently, Drumm *et al.* observed *Helicobacter-like* organisms in 70% of 67 pediatric patients with a chronic-active

Gastritis [4]. Related findings have been made of spiral-shaped species colonizing the mucosa and the overlying gastric-epithelium mucus layer Infiltrate gastric inflammatory cells Czinn and Carrl in 25 children. More studies indicate that *H. pylori* colonization in the gastritis of a primarily chronic inflammatory cell infiltrate is almost always linked to gastritis in children [5, 6]. Reports of *H. pylori* eradication from gastric mucus suggest that the antral gastritis is resolved in combination with a single core case sequence. However, *H. pylori*-infected children have not undergone multicenter randomized controlled eradication trials and are important [6].

Studies in adults established the presence of the organism in nearly all cases of chronic gastritis [7]. At first, *H. pylori* was proposed to colonize inflamed tissue, rather than to induce inflammation, since gastritis is widespread in adults [7]. However, the prevalence of gastritis is less frequent in children thereby enabling the investigation of *H. pylori* as a cause for gastritis rather than an opportunistic colonizer of inflamed tissue [8]. Studies have observed that colonization of *H. pylori* in children with secondary causes, such as NSAID, eosinophilic gastroenteritis and Crohn's disease is not normal in the gastric mucosa [8]. These findings together show clearly the pathogenic role of *H. pylori* in the development of chronic antral gastritis in infants.

For over a century, bacteria have been known to be found in the human body [9]. These bacteria, however, were thought to be contaminants from digested food rather than true gastric colonizers. Around 20 years ago, the isolation and culture of a bacterial spiral species known later as *Helicobacter pylori* was announced successfully by Barry and Robin Warren [10], from the human stomach. Self-ingestion experiments by Marshall [11] and Morris [12] and later experiments with volunteers [13] demonstrated that these bacteria can colonize the human stomach, thereby inducing inflammation of the gastric mucosa. After ingestion of *H. pylori*, Marshall produced intermittent gastritis; Morris' condition progressed into more persistent gastritis, which cleared doxycycline and sub-salicylate bismuth after sequential care. These initial data were closely used as a stimulus in further studies, demonstrating that gastrointestinal disorders such as chronic gastric gastritis, peptic ulcer, lymphoma associated with gastric mucous membrane and stomach cancer can lead to a variety of upper gastrointestinal disorders. This knowledge has a direct therapeutic influence on disease control. In addition, insights into the pathogenesis of chronic disease are provided by the persistence of a pathogen in an area long believed to be sterile. This discovery has resulted in Robin Warren and Barry Marshall's "discovery of the bacterium *Helicobacter pylori* and his role in gastritis and peptic ulcer diseases" won the 2005 Nobel Prize in physiology or medicine.

The genus *Helicobacter* belongs to the subdivision of the *Proteobacteria*, order *Campylobacterales*, family *Helicobacteraceae*. This family also includes the genera *Wolinella*, *Flexispira*, *Sulfurimonas*, *Thiomicrospira*, and *Thiovulum*. The Helicobacter genus consists of more than 20 species, all of which have been recognized officially. Members of the Helicobacter family are all microaerophile organisms and most of them are positive for catalase and oxidase and many but not all species also are positive for urease [14].

It is possible to separate Helicobacter species into two main lines, the gastric helicobacter species and the enterohepatic (nongastric) species of Helicobacter. They have a strong degree of organ specificity, which in general indicates gastric helicobacter cannot colonize the intestine or liver, and vice versa.

2. Gastric *Helicobacter* species

Gastric Helicobacter organisms have evolved to the unfriendly environments at the stomach surface and are currently suspected to colonize the stomachs of all mammals through Helicobacter members. The urease is positive and extremely mobile by flagella are all recognized gastric Helicobacter species [15, 16]. Urease is believed to enable brief survival in a very acidic gastric lumen, but motility has been thought to allow quick travel into the more neutral pH of gastric mucosa; this may explain why the colonization of gastric mucosa is conditional upon both factors [17]. When joining, the Helicobacter gastric species display a chemical motility of urea and bicarbonate to the mucus layer [16]. The spiral morphology and flagellate motility help the viscous mucus layer penetrate, where the more pH-neutral conditions allow the genital Helicobacter species to grow.

i. *Helicobacter felis*

ii. *Helicobacter mustelae*

iii. *Helicobacter acinonychis*

iv. *Helicobacter heilmannii*.

H. pylori is a demanding micro-organism that needs complex media for development. Sometimes, blood or serum was applied to these medias. These supplements are additional food sources and can also be used for defending against long-chain fatty acid toxic effects [18].

H. pylori associated gastritis is characterized by the presence of acute and chronic inflammation, with immature surface epithelial cells [19]. Mucus degeneration is also found by successful cell renewal of epithelial cells. The degree of mucosal infection ranges from the lowest inflammatory infiltration in lamina propria to the extreme gastritis with thick mucoal inflammation with retained architecture. In extreme cases, all surface epithelium and gastric wells can be used as micro-abscesses for intraepithelial neutrophils [20].

Previously, it was believed that in *H. pylori* gastritis, fundic inflammation was less important than that of the antral mucosa [21]. However, *H. pylori* and gastroesophageal reflux disease create, or arise concurrently, may also be caused by the anatomical role of the inflammatory cell infiltrate [22]. Moreover, patients who have been receiving a proton pump inhibitor for acid suppression frequently have colonization of fundic and cardia mucosa by *H. pylori*. Carditis, of both a chronic and active phenotype, is frequent in *H. pylori*-infected adults [23]. Children require research to help establish the association between *H. pylori* infection, gastric inflammation sites and sequalae of long-term diseases.

H. pylori-associated gastritis in children is commonly not apparent at endoscopy, thereby making biopsy essential for definitive diagnosis [24]. Nodularity of the antral mucosa has been described in association with *H. pylori* gastritis in children [25]. Its value has not yet been identified. However, antral nodularity was found in *H. pylori* infected adults and less common in children [26].

Columbia or Brucella agar, (lysed) horse or sheep blood agar, or fetal calf serum as substitute, is widely used as a solid medium for regular isolation and *H. pylori* culture.

3. Transmission and sources of infection

Most unknown are the precise processes by which *H. pylori* is obtained. *H. pylori* has a small host range and is present in people and some non-human primates nearly exclusively.

In rare cases, the presence of pets may be a concern for *H. pylori* infection; hence, pets should be isolated [27]. There is also no definitive proof for zoonotic *H. pylori* transmission [28]. The direct transmission from person to person, either oral or fecal-oral route or both, is expected to lead to new infections. In saliva, vomit, gastric refluxate and diarrhea, *H. pylori* has been detected [29]. Yet there is no definitive proof that either of these products had the predominant transmission. This may be because most transmission research has concentrated on adults.

It indicates that for dentists, gastroenterologist, nurses, spousal partners or physicians with sexually transmitted diseases there was no clear rise in risk of carrying *H. pylori* [30]. As a result of these and other investigations, it is generally believed that acquisition mostly occurs in early childhood, most likely from close family members [31].

Crowding inside and outside families with children are both linked to the occurrence of *H. pylori* [32], Although the adult crowd seems less significant, except for some situations, for example amongst military recruits [33]. Several experiments have shown that *H. pylori* DNA is found in environmental bodies of water [34].

Spread via fecal contaminants is supported by the occurrence of *H. pylori* infections among institutionalized young people during outbreaks of gastroenteritis [35]. Additional sources are infected food, as *H. pylori* can briefly live on cooled food [36]. In tandem with *H. pylori's* intense exposure to oxygen demand, nutrient exclusion and temperatures outside 34–40°C [37]. The most likely path of direct person-to-person transmission.

The incidence of gastric cancer is higher in poor areas and in developing and advanced countries in lower socioeconomic groups [38]. Gastric cancer remains the most prevalent malignancy among men and the second most commonly identified among women in many countries of Latin America and Asia. Colombia and Japan recorded incidence rates of up to 80 per 100,000 populations. The gastric cancer in the United States and Western Europe, by comparison, affects less than 10 per 100,000 individuals per year [39]. However, ethnic groups with elevated risk remain in low-risk nations. For instance, in the US, gastric cancer is nearly double that prevalent among Blacks, Asians and Hispanics. It is noteworthy that *H. pylori* prevalence rates are 2-10 times higher in all of these populations than in the total population [40].

4. Clinical aspects of *H. pylori*-associated diseases

H. pylori colonization is not an infection itself, but it impacts the relative likelihood that multiple pathological conditions of the upper gastrointestinal tract and even the hepatobiliary tract will grow. Therefore, *H. pylori* examination alone is not relevant but can be done in order to ascertain the cause of a basic disorder, such as peptic ulcer disease or to avoid disease, for example in subjects with family gastric carcinoma. A positive test result will validate the procedure, and a negative test result can suggest that other etiological causes or prevention steps needs to be examined.

4.1 Types of Disease

Although gastric *H. pylori* colonization causes histologic gastritis in all infected persons, only a minority experience any apparent clinical symptoms. *H. pylori*-positive patients are estimated to have a 10–20 percent life-cycle risk for ulcer and a 1–2 percent risk for distal gastric cancer [41]. The probability of developing *H. pylori* disorders depends on a range of bacterial, host, and environmental factors, most of which are related to gastritis pattern and severity (**Figure 1**).

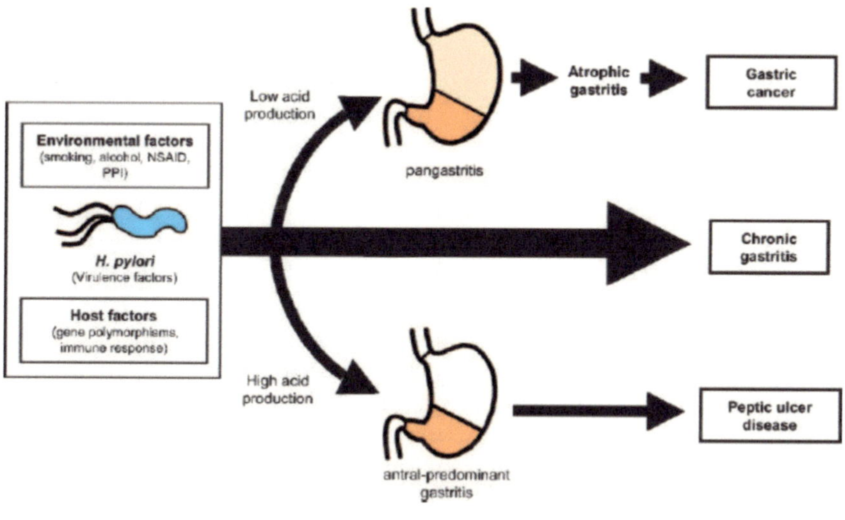

Figure 1.
Schematic representation of the factors contributing to gastric pathology and disease outcome in H. pylori *infection [42].*

4.2 Acute and chronic gastritis

The scale of *H. pylori* colonization nearly always contributes to gastric mucosa invasion of neutrophilic and mononuclear cells in the antrum and corpus. The principal condition of this chronic active gastritis is *H. pylori* colonization, in particular as consequence of this chronic inflammation phase, and other *H. pylori*-related conditions [42].

4.2.1 Acute gastritis

Acute infection results are uncommon and come mostly from accounts of subjects who knowingly or accidentally took *H. pylori* or were exposed to hazardous substance procedures [43]. Recently, an *H. pylori* infection human challenge model was introduced, which permitted managed acute infection analysis with deliberate safe volunteer infection by a well-characterized *H. pylori* laboratory strain [44]. Along with these findings, these reports have shown that the acute process of *H. pylori* colonization can include temporary non-specific dyspeptic symptoms, including completeness, nausea, vomiting, and severe inflammation of the proximal, and distal stomach mucus or pangastritis. This process is also related to the period of months of hypochlorhydria. It is uncertain whether spontaneous clearing and resolution of gastritis can be accompanied by this initial colonization and, if so, how often that happens. Further trials in young children with serology or breathing tests have shown that certain patients in this age group might spontaneously lose the infection [45]; This was not found in the development of atrophic gastritis other than under particular circumstances.

Studies of homozygotic twins however demonstrated a concordance with their classification as *H. pylori* regardless of their cohabitation or break [46]. This consensus between heterozygous twins has not been observed. This indicates that some people are likely to be colonized with *H. pylori* while others may avoid or eradicate a proven infection. This theory is also backed by the finding that *H. pylori* sensitivity in many developing countries is very strong in young age and yet chronic *H. pylori* infections are never acquired by any individuals.

4.2.2 Chronic gastritis

When colonization becomes persistent, the acid secretion level and the gastritis distribution interact closely (**Figure 2**). The association between acid and bacterial growth arises from the counteractive effects of acid against bacterial growth and subsequent mutation inflammation on the acid separation and regulation. The effect of *H. pylori* infection is important in this relationship. *H. pylori* particularly colonizes the gastric antrum in subjects with intact acid secretion, where there are only a few parietal acid secretory cells present [42].

This pattern of colonization is linked to gastritis which prevails. Histological examination of the gastric corpus specimens shows that the amount of superficially colonized *H. pylori* bacteria is reduced by chronically dormant inflammation and that. Those of which the secretion of acid is affected by some process have a more equal distribution of bacteria in the antrum and corpus and are in closer proximity of the mucosa bacteria, inducing pangastritis, which are predominate [47].

The acid secretion may be diminished by loss of parietal cells due to atrophic gastritis, but it can also happen when acid's secretive potential is intact, although the work of parietal cells is inhibited by vagotomy or acid-suppressive drugs, particularly proton pump inhibitors (PPIs) [47]. The subsequent active inflammation of the corpses raises hypochlorhydra parallel to an acute period of infection with a strong suppressive effect on the celestial function, since local inflammatory factors, including cytokines, like interleukin-1 beta (IL-1 β) are strongly suppressive. Different findings illustrate that. The first argument is that *H. pylori*-corpus gastritis frequently is related to hypochlorhydrate, and eradication treatment leads to greater secretion of acid [48].

Secondly, *H. pylori* corpus gastritis augments the acid-suppressive effects of PPIs [49]. As a result, *H. pylori*-positive patients with gastroesophageal reflux disease (GERD) may respond somewhat faster to PPI treatment both with respect to symptom resolution and with healing of esophagitis [50], However, this effect of everyday clinical practice is marginal and essentially negligible. This means that the status of *H. pylori* is not general in decision-making regarding GERD dose of PPI medication. A third observation in favor of the acid repression effects of active corpus gastritis has been made in more recent significant research that indicates the risk of corpus predominant pangastritis from subject with proinflammatory genotype predisposing people to atrophic gastritis, intestinal metaplasia and gastric cancer [51].

Pattern of gastritis	*Gastric histology*	*Duodenal histology*	*Acid secretion*	*Clinical condition*
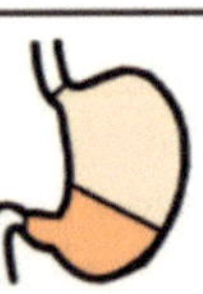 Pan-gastritis	• Chronic inflammation • Atrophy • Intestinal metaplasia	• Normal	• Reduced	• Gastric ulcer • Gastric cancer
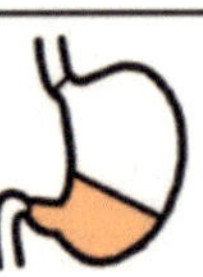 Antral-predominant	• Chronic inflammation • Polymorph activity	• Gastric metaplasia • Active chronic inflammation	• Increased	• Duodenal ulcer

Figure 2.
Acid secretion and the associated pattern of gastritis play an important role in disease outcome in H. pylori *infection. The figure displays the correlations between the pattern of* H. pylori *colonization, inflammation, acid secretion, gastric and duodenal histology, and clinical outcome [42].*

Although colonization by *H. pylori* is almost invariably associated with gastritis, and gastritis is mainly attributed to colonization by *H. pylori*, gastritis is due to other causes of gastritis, such as cytomegalovirus, chronic inflammatory idiopathic diseases, and auto-immune disease such as Crohn's disease and pernicious anemia.

5. Role of *H. pylori* virulence factors

5.1 *cag* PAI (Pathogenicity Island)

Although the *H. pylori* infection nearly always triggers chronic active gastritis, most affected patients are free of apparent health signs and have no other complications [52]. This lead to the belief that some strains could be more virulent than others. Early studies of variations of *H. pylori* strains demonstrated the capacity of such virulent strains to cause morphological changes, vacuolizations and successive degeneration from in vitro-cultivated cells. This pathogenicity is linked [53]. This activity was then linked to the presence of a protein with a molecular mass of approximately 140 kDa that was named CagA (for "cytotoxinassociated gene A").

The CagA protein is a highly immunogenic protein encoded by the *cagA* gene [54]. About 50–70 percent of *H. pylori* strains have this gene [55] and is a marker for the presence of a genomic PAI of about 40 kb that, depending on the strain analyzed, encodes between 27 and 31 proteins [54]. Strains carrying the Cag PAI are called CagA+ strains, as their ability to cause major antibody titers against the CagA marker protein is widely recognized in patients. In CagA patients, inflammation is typically higher and the probability of developing a signs (peptic ulcer or gastric cancer) in western populations is considerably higher [56], though not in Asian populations [57]. While CagA+ strains are associated with a higher risk of ulceration, gastritis and gastric cancer, cag PAI strains are also associated with a higher risk of peptic ulcer or gastrointestinal cancer, even though at a smaller frequency.

Eighteen cag PAI-coded proteins are used to form a type IV secretive unit that forms a structure like a syringe that is able to penetrate gastric epithelial cells and to promote the translocation of CagA, peptidoglycan, and probably other bacterial components into host cells [58] (**Figure 3**). Once delivered inside the cell, the CagA protein is phosphorylated at tyrosine residues in EPIYA motifs [59] by Src family kinases [60]. Phosphorylated CagA interacted then with a number of host signaling molecules, including tyrosine phosphate SHP-2, which results in morphological changes in the epithelial cells [61].

Apoptosis of T cells is impaired by the cag PAI since the immune response is also affected [62]. The association of type IV formation with the host cell also results in pro-inflammatory cytokines in epithelial cell induction [63].

It was originally believed that this proinflammatory cytokines are caused by a CagA protein itself, but nowadays CagA only plays, if any, a minor role in triggering them [63]. It is possible that the intimate contact with the IV-type form contributes to peptidoglycan leak into the eukaryotic cell [64] (**Figure 3**), although it cannot be ruled out completely that the activation of the IL-8 signaling cascade results from the translocation of a thus-far-unknown bacterial factor [63].

Tyrosine Phosphorylation is necessary for binding CagA to SHP-2 within the CagA EPIYA motif. [65]. The number of EPIYA tyrosine phosphorylation motives within the CagA proteins of various *H. pylori* isolates varies considerably. CagA is specifically correlated with the amount of repetitions of tyrosine phosphorylation. [66]. Strains with a larger number of CagA repetitions cause more marked morphological changes in cultivated epithelial cells [67] and an increased risk of gastric carcinogenesis being correlated. CagA also interacts through SH2 domains with the

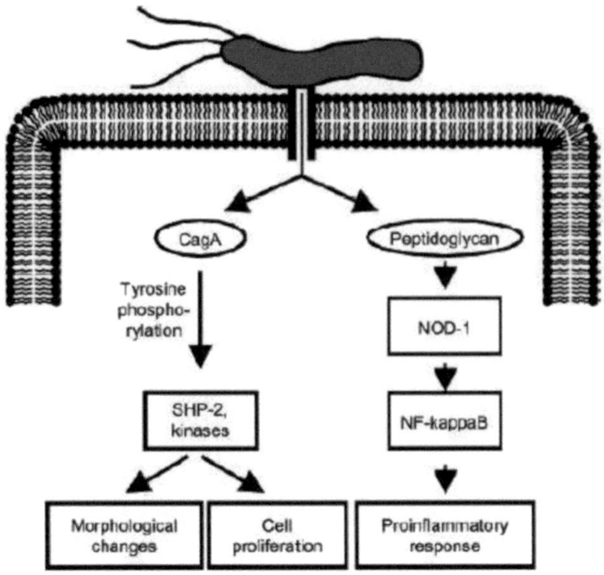

Figure 3.
Schematic representation of the different roles of the Cag type IV secretion system in immune modulation, cell proliferation, and morphological changes [42].

c-terminal Src kinase, which contributes to c-tyrosine Src's kinase inactivation. This inactivation, since it mediates CagA tyrosine phosphorylation, leads to a decrease in CagA phosphorylation, thereby creating a feedback loop to control CagA behavior [65]. This cross talk of host-pathogen results in tested virulence and can thus serve to colonize the host for a lifetime.

5.2 VacA vacuolating cytotoxin

Around 50% of all strains of *H. pylori* secrete VacA, a highly immunogenic 95 kDa protein that is causing massive vacuolisation of epithel cells in vitro [68]. VacA is a key factor in both peptic ulceration and gastric cancer pathogenesis. Though VacA is not necessary for in vitro growth of *H. pylori* the murine gastric colonization by *H. pylori* has been shown to make a substantial contribution [69].

The activities of VacA include development of the membrane channel, endosomal and lysosomal disorders, incorporate cell receptor signaling effects and cytoskeleton-related interference with cell-dependent functions, apoptosis induction and immune regulation (**Figure 4**). Although vacuolization is readily observed in vitro, it does not seem to occur *in vivo* [42]. The VacA protein is formed with a protoxin of 140 kDa and is broken into the shape of 95 kDa as it is secreted.

While all strains have a functional vacA gene, the vacuolating activities among strains differ considerably [69]. This is due to the sequence heterogeneity within the *vacA* gene at the signal region (s) and the middle region (m). The s region of the gene, which encodes the signal peptide, occurs as either an s1 or s2 type, whereas the m region, which contains the p58 cell binding domain, exists as an m1 or m2 type [70].

In the cell epithelial membrane, VacA forms pores that cause urea and anions to be released from the host cells. It also enhances transcellular penetration, resulting in nutrient and cation releases [71]. Interestingly, a major portion of the secreted toxin does not go to the environment, but is bound to the outer membrane of *H. pylori*. These toxin clusters are passed to the host cell surface following bacterial

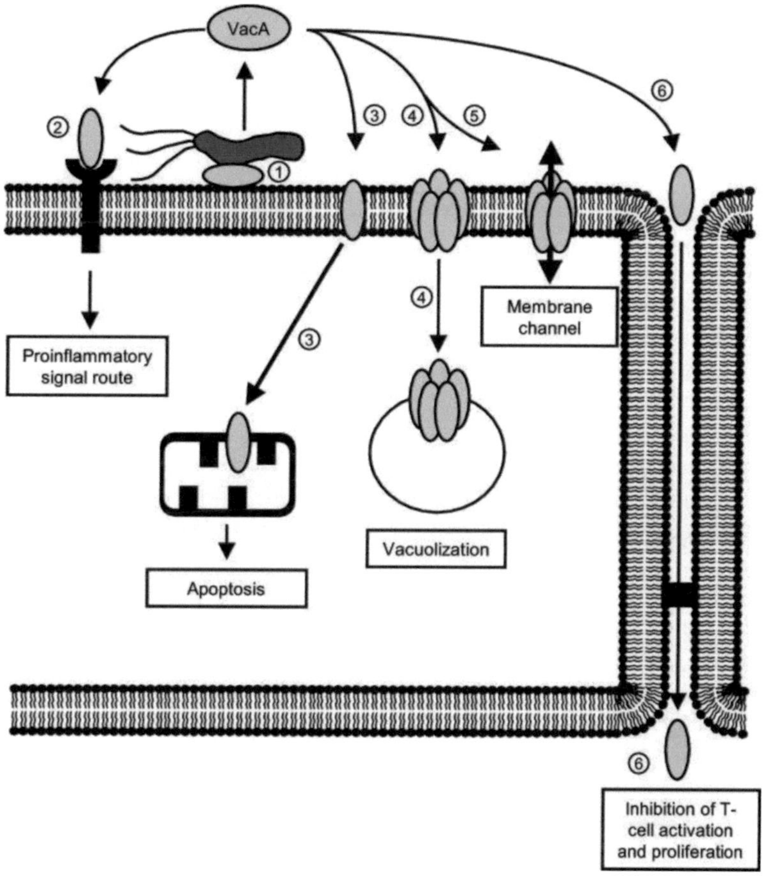

Figure 4.
The VacA protein influences cellular processes via different routes, thus assisting in chronic colonization of the gastric mucosa by H. pylori. *(1) Surface-bound VacA may be directly delivered to the cell membrane. Secreted VacA may either (2) bind to a cell membrane receptor and initiate a proinflammatory response, (3) be taken up directly by the cell and be trafficked to the mitochondria and induce apoptosis, (4) be taken up by pinocytosis and induce vacuolization, (5) form a membrane channel, resulting in leakage of nutrients to the extracellular space, or (6) pass through the tight junctions and inhibit T-cell activation and proliferation. (Modified with permission from* Nature Reviews Microbiology *[23].*

interaction with their host cells and have their toxic effects. This touch-dependent mechanism for direct delivery proposes the inclusion in bacterial-cell contact of particular receptors. However, such a receptor has not yet been identified [72].

Secreted VacA can be further processed into a 33-kDa N-terminal fragment and a 55-kDa C-terminal fragment through proteolytic cleavage. In the development of anion channels, the N-terminal protein plays an important role while C-terminal proteins mediate cell binding [73].

In spite of the proteolytic cleavage, these fragments remain noncovalently associated with each other [74]. Spontaneously purified VacA forms oligomeric aggregates and disassembles in the active monomers of pores in the cell membrane after exposed to acidic pH. Spontaneously purified VacA forms oligomeric aggregates and disassembles in the active monomers of pores in the cell membrane after exposed to acidic pH but are likely to be an *in vitro* artifact [75].

While several VacA-mediated effects are induced by membrane binding and pore formation, VacA also reaches the cytosol, then accumulates in the mitochondrial inner membrane and causes apoptosis, activating endogenous mitochondrial channels [76]. The proapoptotic influence of VacA is based on the cell type and may be restricted to gastric epithelial cells like parietal cells. This may result in reduced acid secretion, thereby predisposing for development of gastric cancer [77].

6. Pathogenesis of infection

6.1 *H. pylori*-associated pathogenesis

Chronic active gastritis is the principal disease after *H. pylori* colonization. In all *H. pylori*-positive subjects this syndrome can be found. Various different factors such as colonizing stress characteristics, host physiology, immune response, diet, and development rate depend on the intragastric distribution and intensity of the chronic inflammatory process. Many of the complications of this chronic inflammation include *H. pylori*-induced ulcers, gastric cancer and lymphoma; in particular, ulcerative and gastric cancers arise in these people and in the areas of the most serious inflammation. Therefore, recognizing these factors is important in order to consider *H. pylori's* role in the etiology of the upper gastrointestinal disorder [42].

H. pylori colonizes the membrane in the stomach antrum of the gastric epithelia. *H. pylori* adhere to the stomach epithelia is a prime and significant step towards colonization of gastric mucosa and gastritis [78].

In duodenum, *H. pylori* only infects gastric mucosa and gastric metaplasia [79]. In comparison, on intestinal epithelium *H. pylori* is never seen. Dunn *et al.*, stated in vitro, that *H. pylori* was more effective than human intestine (Int-407) cells, and sac cells with yolk bags, on human gastric epithelial cells [80]. Similarly, the adherence rate of *H. pylori* to gastric cell lines (KatoIII, MKN45) was shown to be significantly higher than that to Int-407 cells. These results indicate that *H. pylori* has specific binding activity to human gastric epithelial cells [81].

In a logarithmic point, *H. pylori* has strong nourishment with a spiral morphology. But spiral to coccoid conversion may be inducted by alkaline pH, rise in temperature, antibiotic therapy, aerobics or anaerobics, or prolonged incubation. The type of coccoid *H. pylori* is known as viable but not cultivable. *H. pylori* coccoid bind to both the stomach epithelial MKN45 cells and the spiral form. Although it is unknown whether the coccoid form has any role in the infection pathogenesis., Cole *et al.*" The type of coccoid has been reported to bind badly to gastric epithelial cells. In contrast to spiral shape the form induces a short interleukin 8 (IL-8) chain. The coccoid shape, by comparison, was more frequent than the spiral of *H. pylori* induces cellular changes of pedestal formation [82].

6.2 Gastric environment at the site of infection

The human stomach has a medium luminal pH, with elevations until around pH 4 during meals due to nutrient buffering, when set to natural physiological acid secretion [83]. *H. pylori* originally occupied a more neutral niche at the gastric region with gastric acidity defense offered by the secretion of bicarbonate from epithelial cells and mucus. Studies with glass microelectrodes indicated a pH gradient in the stomach mucus and an epithelial pH virtually neutral [84]. The measuring technique may have delayed these studies as open tip microelectrodes may have stopped proton diffusion. Later microelectrode experiments using a similar method of calculation in mice found that all obstacles to the proton diffusion were eliminated and acidic pH was indicated in the bacterial niche [85]. Fluorescent dyeing tests in the anesthetic mice's externalized stomachs showed an acidic gastral pH surface regardless of the mucus layer [86]. The pH of the gastric surface is a combination between the regulation of acid and alkaline secretion at a certain stage instead of the trapping of mucus-layer buffers or protons [87].

Analysis of *H. pylori* transcriptome provides additional evidence of acidic pH on gastric surfaces. Several in Vitro experiments have reported improvements in acidic pH expression of the gene using varying duration and conditions of incubation [87–89]. The unifying finding of these research studies is that there are a variety of genes that alter expression depending on environmental pH and indicate adaptation in order to permit gastric colonization.

The well-documented movements of *H. pylori* from its usual gastric niche to the fundus in human or gerbil acid inhibitory Therapy are proof that the bacteria need to remain in a particular pH setting [90–92]. The *H. pylori* transcriptome has been studied in the gerbil's stomach to correlate with in vitro pH changes [93]. Gerbil is a suitable model system since the gastric pH profile of *H. pylori* and its advanced sequelae are close to the ones found in humans [94–96]. The pattern of *H. pylori* gene changes in the gerbil stomach were comparable to gene changes seen in vitro at acidic pH, providing additional evidence for an acidic environment at the site of infection [97].

6.3 Attaching and effacement by adherence of *H. pylori*

Attaching and effacement is characterized by microvilli effacement, actin rearrangement and pedestal formation following bacterial adhesion to cells as described for enteropathogenic *Escherichia coli* (EPEC) [7]. The attachment and effacement of *H. pylori* in the gastric cells have been documented [97].

The tyrosine Phosphorylation of two host cell proteins (145 kDa and 105 kDa) has been shown to be inducted after *H. pylori* binding to gastric pathologic cells. Although it is hypothesized that tyrosine Phosphoryphorylation of host cell proteins is implicated in pathogenesis of gastric diseases related to *H. pylori* infection However, other researchers found that an attachment of *H. pylori* does not contribute to pedestal formation or actin rearrangement [98].

6.4 Adhesin of *H. pylori* and its receptor

H. pylori adhesively adheres to a receptor on the gastric cell surface by its adhesives. The adhesins and their receivers have been recorded in several respects. As the adhesion of *H. pylori* to cells is not entirely hindered by the human antibody to an adhesin, adherence by the use of many adhesins and their receptors is known to be the outcome.

6.5 HpaA (Sialyllactose-Binding Adhesin)

Evans *et al.* to purified 20 kDa protein as an adhesin of *H. pylori* recognizing N-acetylneuraminyllactose, and cloned its gene, *hpaA*. The protein HpaA functions as hemagglutinin and aggregates the fibrillary structure together. HpaA is stated to be a lipoprotein intracellular and the inactivation of the HpaA did not affect *H. pylori's* adherence to gastric cells. Consequently, the value of HpaA as *H. pylori* adhesin is contentious [99].

6.6 Adhesin recognizing phosphatidylethanolaurine

Specific binding of *H. pylori* to a glycerophospholipid species in the antrum of the human stomach was reported. The thin-layer chromatogram overlay technique showed this species to be a type of phosphatidylethanolamine. Since the exoenzyme from *Pseudomonas aeruginosa* displays similar binding specificity, the binding of *H. pylori* to its lipid receptor was expected to be induced by an exoenzyme S-like adhesive [100].

6.7 BabA protein recognizing Lewisb antigen

The lewis antigens (Lewis, Lewisb, Lewisx, and LewisY) are one of the blood-group antigens that is flucosylated and expressed in human epithelics and erythrocytes. Lewis antigen that recognizes non-secretory blood groups (O) has been reported to be mediating adhesion of *H. pylori* to human gastric epithelial cells. Preferential relation between *H. pylori* and Lewisb antigen suggests that certain patients are more vulnerable to the development of peptic ulcers [101].

6.8 Adhesin recognizing extracellular matrix components

Many researchers have reported that *H. pylori* has been bound to different extracellular matrix components such as vitronectin, heparin sulfate, collagen, fibronectin, lactoferrin, plasminogen and laminin. There are about 20 Specific attachment of *H. pylori* to extracellular matrix components promotes bacterial colonization [102].

6.9 Induction of secretion of various cytokines from gastric cells

In vivo, *H. pylori* gastric infection induces several cytokines, including IL–l beta, IL–6, IL-7 and alpha tumor necrosis, to develop mucous membranes. IL-8 particularly consists of a small peptide (chemokine), secreted by a range of cell types, which helps to attract and activate neutrophils as a powerful inflammatory mediator. IL-8 development stimulation in gastric epithelial cells was recorded by *H. pylori*. The positive CagA strains displayed a significant increase in IL-8 relative to cag negative strains. Transposon inactivation of several genes in *cagA* pathogenicity island (PAl) showed that various genes *(cagB)* C) *D) E)* G) *H, ~ L) A1)* were responsible for the induction of IL-8 from gastric epithelial cells [29]. Recently, Li et al., [30] reported that multiple genes encoding HP052l, 0525, 0527, 0528 and 0529 ORF in the left half of the *cag* PAl of *H. pylori* are required for tyrosine-kinase dependent transcription of IL-8 in gastric epithelial cells. In addition, Yamaguchi et al., [31] reported the induction of IL-8 by HSP60 of *H. pylori* from gastric epithelial KatoIII cells [103].

7. *H. pylori* gastritis and the possible pathogenic

7.1 Role of anti-gastric autoimmune reactions

The serological study in *H. pylori* gastritis provided more indications on the relation between anti gastric autoimmunity and *H. pylori* gastritis. In older patients, *H. pylori* infection is linked to developing anti-parietal cell antibodies [55]. In addition, some *H. pylori*-infected patients, observed 32 years, produce both chronic atrophic gastritis and anti-parietal cell antibodies [104]. These patients eventually become *H. pylori* negative. Also Negrini *et al.*, reported on autoantibodies against gastric epithelial cells in up to 84% of *H. pylori* infected subjects [105].

When sera of *H. pylori-infected* subjects were screened for autoantibodies reacting against human gastric tissue by immunohistochemistry, for these autoantibodies two separate binding sites could be seen; The luminal membranes in the antral and corpus mucosa foveolar epithelial cells first and the channel membranes in the gastric corpus mucosa, second in the parietal cells. Antichannel autoanticorps were called the latter type [106].

7.2 Motility

In early childhood, *H. pylori* infection is obtained through oral-oral or oral-fecal infection. The microbe has to enter its chosen location of colonization, the mucosa of the gastric antrum in the first phase towards colonization. *H. pylori* has formed a spiral mode and unipolar scourge to enter the gastric niche to transit the mucus membrane that overlays the gastric epithelial surface. Host factors steer the migration of *H. pylori* towards the gastric mucosa by means of the chemical reaction of bacteria.

The transcription from intracellular localized components to extracellular flagellar filaments is transient regulated by the expression of the flagellar gene. *H. pylori* is primarily present on the usual acid-secreting stomach, with about one-third of the mucus layer next to the epithelial cells (0–5 μm) in a predominant 15–30 μm mucus above the antrum [107]. About 2 percent of bacteria bind to the gastric epithelium. In order to colonize this niche, the bacteria find that the host attractants or repellents and travel toward or away from them, respectively.

Urea, bicarbonate, pH, zinc, nickel, arginine, glutamine, histidine, and other amino acids elicit chemotactic responses by *H. pylori* [108–112]. These chemotactic factors are sensed by methylaccepting chemotaxis proteins (MCPs) that transduce the signal and alter flagellar rotation. *H. pylori* has at least four MCPs, the membrane proteins TlpA, TlpB, and TlpC and the cytoplasm located TlpD. TlpA senses arginine, other amino acids, and bicarbonate [108]; TlpB is required for pH and urea taxis and also senses the quorum sensing molecule autoinducer- 2 (AI-2) [113]; TlpC regulates whether acid is sensed as an attractant or repellent [111]; and TlpD senses the internal energy state of the bacterium [114].

7.3 Acid acclimation

Colonization is prevented by gastric acid. *H. pylori* is a neutrophil that rises from pH 6.0 to 8.0 and lives from pH 4.0 to 8.0. Since the median pH of the stomach is less than 2.0 and *H. pylori* not only lives in this high acidity, but also prospers, the single acid acclimation process has evolved. The ability of *H. pylori* to retain a near-neutral periplasmic pH in an acidic environment is accurate [115]. This is different from the acid resistance mechanism which enables a cytoplasmic pH near 5 to allow bacteria to transit the stomach [116]. Examples of proteins involved with acid resistance include the glutamate decarboxylase- glutamate aminobutyrate antiporter and the arginine decarboxylase-arginineagmatine antiporter, which consume protons and produce carbon dioxide, and the proton transporters including the F 1 F 0 ATPase and the Na +/2H + antiporter [117, 118]. These systems are designed to control the cytoplasm but do not monitor the pH of periplasm.

Gastric colonization is not possible if cytoplasmic pH cannot be elevated to a level that allows critical metabolic processes such as protein synthesis, a level of buffering that requires periplasmic pH regulation [116]. While *H. pylori* expresses some of the known acid resistance or tolerance genes [119], these proteins complement rather than explain gastric colonization. The principle component of acid acclimation is the neutral pH optimum, highly expressed cytoplasmic urease enzyme. The *H. pylori* urease gene cluster is made up of seven genes under the control of two promoters. *ureA* and *ureB*, under the control of the first promoter, encode the structural subunits of the urease enzyme [120].

Urease is a hexameric heterodimer that requires nickel incorporation for activation. Downstream from the second promoter are *ureI*, *ureE*, *ureF*, *ureG*, and *ureH* [121]. *ureI* encodes in an operon the only integral membrane protein. The Cytoplasmic proteins *UreE, UreF, UreG, and UreH* help to integrate nickel in apourease.

Urease is required for acid survival and gastric colonization [122, 123]. *H. pylori* urease production is constitutive, contributing about 10 percent of the total cell protein [124, 125]. A neutral pH-based cytoplasmic enzyme catalyzes the degradation of urea into carbonic acid and, eventually. With a low pH activity and inactivation, the pH-reduced into the region contained inside the intestines, the activity curve of the free urease is optimum near neutral. The activity of urease in intact bacteria is marginal at neutral pH and increases to no more than pH 6 to roughly pH 2.5 [126]. This curve of activity indicates a limit to urea entry to the enzyme. The only membrane protein of the urease gene cluster, UreI, was seen as a proton gated urea channel, which enables urea into cytoplasm at acidic pH [127]. Deletion of *ureI* leads to loss of acid activation of urease [125]. ureI deletion mutants cannot live in acid at physiologic urea concentrations. Periplasmic pH sinks as well as the medium pH drops. This leads to opening of UreI, movement of urea into the cytoplasm, and breakdown to the eventual end products of carbon dioxide and ammonia, catalyzed by the urease enzyme. The two gasses then buffer the periplasm to the pH range that is consistent with neutrophil survival without having to adjust the atmosphere with bulk pH.

Ni 2+ per active site are required for activation of urease, and a large fraction of urease can be inactive, especially at neutral pH [128, 129]. This will likely avoid the over-alkalization of this neutrophil in situations where the pH increases, and would thus create a urease pool that is primed and ready to go into action in setting a decrease in pH [130]. UreE forms a heterodimer with UreG and UreF with UreH, as evidenced by yeast two hybrid and homology analysis, and these protein pairs bind urease most likely via UreB to aid with nickel incorporation and enzyme activation [131, 132]. Each accessory protein has a specific role in urease activation. UreE aids directly with incorporation of nickel into the active site [132]. UreF prevents premature nickel binding [133]. UreG provides energy for assembly of urease. UreH provides stability for apourease [134]. A broad number of regulatory mechanisms, many of which are involved in acid survival, can be controlled directly and indirected by the nickel regulation protein NikR [135]. For example, NikR has been shown both in vitro and in vivo to positively regulate expression of *ureA* [136–139].

7.4 pH alteration and treatment efficacy

H. pylori is unique for survival in an acidic gastric environment, but bacteria are separated and formed at neutral pH as a neutrophil. Transcription of growth-dependent genes in higher medium pH is increased [140]. Most antibiotics used in treating *H. pylori* infection are bacterial-dependent for optimum effectiveness. Ampicillin is slightly more effective at near-neutral pH against *H. pylori* in vitro [140]. Adding bismuth to the treatment regimens also has a pH effect, at least in part, because the compound impairs the proton entry and reduces the decrease in cytoplasmic pH with medium acidification, which improves bacterial metabolism and increased antibiotic effectiveness [141]. With this in mind, The more bacteria are separated in the therapeutic cycle, the more successful conventional treatment, a proton pump inhibitor and a triple or quadruple therapy regimen of antibiotics are used. This concept is likely homologous to the concept of persisters seen across bacterial species.

Persisters are members of a bacterial population that survive exposure to bactericidal antibiotics yet, when re-cultured, display the same antibiotic sensitivity as the population as a whole [142, 143]. *H. pylori* that are not dividing at administered at antibiotic time will not be eliminated, leaving a limited population of viable bacteria that can restore stomach colonization when antibiotics are stopped. At recommended doses, drugs currently available in acid blockade will not achieve the required sustained pH shift to imitate the bactericidal effect seen in in vitro studies [140, 144].

The current treatment effectiveness challenges can be solved by introducing non antibiotic treatment schemes, using the colonization mechanisms mentioned here, by prevention, intervention or acclimatization of motility, adhesion or acidity. The in vitro efficacy of the carbonic anhydrase inhibitor acetazolamide against *H. pylori* is one example of a potential treatment targeting acid acclimation and periplasmic pH regulation [123]. In the creation of new and better treatment regimes, a continuous research and understanding of the molecular processes of *H. pylori* gastric colonization are crucial.

8. Immune response role of antibodies in protective immunity

Analogy with other mucosal pathogens was originally thought to be primarily antibodies to mediate a defensive immune reaction against *H. pylori*. Subsequent studies found that the importance of the humoral immunity mechanism is negligible. Antibodies can prevent infection successfully and decrease the colonization in animal models studies [145]. *H. pylori* infection results in an induction of a Th1-polarized response that does not result, however, in clearance of the infection. This is striking, because the primary function in sterilizing Immunity is stated to be cellular rather than humoral immunity [146], Although it is now widely agreed that *H. pylori*-induced gastritis and/or pathology primarily rely on Th1 cells and Th1 cytokines [147]. While a polarized Th2 reaction defends against this pathology, it doesn't generally include the defense of Th2 cells after immunization. In fact, Th1-polarized T cells recruit mononuclear cells to the infection site instead of Th2-polarized, thereby removing bacteria [148].

9. Conclusion

From various studies it is concluded that gastritis still pose world -wide burden and requires extensive studies on the pathogenesis of the disease. *H. pylori* remains the most causative agent and it possess the virulence factors such as cag pathogenicity island and vacA vacuolating cytotoxin. These factors influence cellular processes via different routes, thus assisting in chronic colonization of the gastric mucosa by *H. pylori*. Gastritis infection highly results in induction of the protective immune response. Further studies should focus on the immunity to gastritis and the role of cytokines should be ruled out.

Author details

Karam Dawood[1*] and Israa Mamdooh[2]

1 Genetic Engineering, Al-Esraa University College, Iraq

2 Microbiology, Al-Esraa University College, Iraq

*Address all correspondence to: karam.dawood@esraa.edu.iq

References

[1] Warren. R., and Marshall B., 1983, Unidentified curved bacilli on gastric epithelium in active chronic gastritis. *Lancet. 1:1273-1275.*

[2] Hill R., Pearman]., Worthy P, Caruso V, Goodwin S., and Blincow E., 1986, *Campylobacter pyloridis* and gastritis in children [letter]. *Lancet. 1(8477):387.*

[3] Cadranel S., Goossens H., De Boeck M., Malengreau A., Rodesch P, and Butzler P, 1986, *Campylobacter pyloridis* in children [letter]. *Lancet. 1(8483):735-736.*

[4] Drumm B., O'Brien A, Cutz E., and Sherman P, 1987, *Campylobacter pyloridis*-associated primary gastritis in children. *Pediatrics.* 80(2): 192-195.

[5] Kilbridge PM., Dahms B. B., and Czinn S, 1988, *Campylobacter pylori*-associated gastritis and peptic ulcer disease in children. *Am. Dis. Child.* 142(11): 1149-1152.

[6] Yeung C. K., Fu K. H., Yuen K. Y, *et al.,* 1990, *Helicobacter pylori* and associated duodenal ulcer. *Arch. Dis. Child.* 65(11): 12121216.

[7] Peterson W. L., 1991, *Helicobacter pylori* and peptic ulcer disease. *N. Engl. Med.* 324(15): 1043-1048.

[8] Drumm B., Sherman P, Cutz E., and Karmali M., 1987, Association of *Campylobacter pylori* on the gastric mucosa with antral gastritis in children. *N. Engl. Med. 316(25):1557-1561.*

[9] Bizzozero, G. 1893. Ueber die schlauchfö rmigen Drü sen des Magendarmkanals und die Beziehungen ihres Epithels zu dem Oberflä chenepithel der Schleimhaut. Dritte mitteilung. Archiv Mikroskopische Anat. 43:82-152.

[10] Warren, J. R., and B. J. Marshall. 1983. Unidentified curved bacilli on gastric epithelium in active chronic gastritis. Lancet i:1273-1275.

[11] Marshall, B. J., J. A. Armstrong, D. B. McGechie, and R. J. Glancy. 1985. Attempt to fulfil Koch's postulates for pyloric *Campylobacter*. Med. J. Austr. 142:436-439.

[12] Morris, A., and G. Nicholson. 1987. Ingestion of *Campylobacter pyloridis* causes gastritis and raised fasting gastric pH. Am. J. Gastroenterol. *82*:192-199.

[13] Morris, A. J., M. R. Ali, G. I. Nicholson, G. I. Perez-Perez, and M. J. Blaser. 1991. Long-term follow-up of voluntary ingestion of Helicobacter pylori. Ann. Intern. Med. 114:662-663.

[14] Fox, J. G. 2002. The non-*H. pylori* helicobacters: their expanding role in gastrointestinal and systemic diseases. Gut 50:273-283.

[15] Solnick, J. V., and D. B. Schauer. 2001. Emergence of diverse *Helicobacter* species in the pathogenesis of gastric and enterohepatic diseases. Clin. Microbiol. Rev. 14:59-97.

[16] Yoshiyama, H., and T. Nakazawa. 2000. Unique mechanism of *Helicobacter pylori* for colonizing the gastric mucus. Microbes Infect. 2:55-60.

[17] Schreiber, S., M. Konradt, C. Groll, P. Scheid, G. Hanauer, H. O. Werling, C. Josenhans, and S. Suerbaum. 2004. The spatial orientation of *Helicobacter pylori* in the gastric mucus. Proc. Natl. Acad. Sci. USA 101:5024-5029.

[18] Taneera, J., A. P. Moran, S. O. Hynes, H. O. Nilsson, W. Al-Soud, and T. Wadstrom. 2002. Influence of activated charcoal, porcine gastric mucin and beta-cyclodextrin on the morphology and growth of intestinal

and gastric Helicobacter spp. Microbiology 148:677-684.

[19] Bury-Mone, S., S. Skouloubris, C. Dauga, J. M. Thiberge, D. Dailidiene, D. E. Berg, A. Labigne, and H. De Reuse. 2003. Presence of active aliphatic amidases in *Helicobacter* species able to colonize the stomach. Infect. Immun. 71:5613-5622.

[20] Bruggraber, S. F., G. French, R. P. Thompson, and J. J. Powell. 2004. Selective and effective bactericidal activity of the cobalt (II) cation against *Helicobacter pylori*. Helicobacter 9: 422-428.

[21] Court, M., P. A. Robinson, M. F. Dixon, and J. E. Crabtree. 2002. Gastric *Helicobacter* species infection in murine and gerbil models: comparative analysis of effects of *H. pylori* and *H. felis* on gastric epithelial cell proliferation. J. Infect. Dis. 186:1348-1352.

[22] Cover, T. L. 1996. The vacuolating cytotoxin of *Helicobacter pylori*. Mol. Microbiol. 20:241-246.

[23] Cover, T. L., and S. R. Blanke. 2005. Helicobacter pylori VacA, a paradigm for toxin multifunctionality. Nat. Rev. Microbiol. 3:320-332.

[24] Contreras, M., J. M. Thiberge, M. A. Mandrand-Berthelot, and A. Labigne. 2003. Characterization of the roles of NikR, a nickel-responsive pleiotropic autoregulator of Helicobacter pylori. Mol. Microbiol. 49:947-963.

[25] Cover, T. L., and M. J. Blaser. 1992. Purification and characterization of the vacuolating toxin from *Helicobacter pylori*. J. Biol. Chem. 267:10570-10575.

[26] Cover, T. L., U. S. Krishna, D. A. Israel, and R. M. Peek, Jr. 2003. Induction of gastric epithelial cell apoptosis by *Helicobacter pylori* vacuolating cytotoxin. Cancer Res. 63:951-957.

[27] Herbarth, O., P. Krumbiegel, G. J. Fritz, M. Richter, U. Schlink, D. M. Muller, and T. Richter. 2001. Helicobacter pylori prevalences and risk factors among school beginners in a German urban center and its rural county. Environ. Health Perspect. 109:573-577.

[28] Fox, J. G. 1995. Nonhuman reservoirs of *Helicobacter pylori*. Aliment. Pharmacol. Ther. 9(Suppl. 2):93-103.

[29] Sinha, S. K., B. Martin, B. D. Gold, Q. Song, M. Sargent, and C. N. Bernstein. 2004. The incidence of *Helicobacter pylori* acquisition in children of a Canadian First Nations community and the potential for parentto- child transmission. Helicobacter 9:59-68.

[30] Me'graud, F. 1995. Transmission of *Helicobacter pylori:* faecal-oral versus oral-oral. Aliment. Pharmacol. Ther. 9:85-91.

[31] van der Ende, A., E. A. J. Rauws, M. Feller, C. J. J. Mulder, G. N. J. Tytgat, and J. Dankert. 1996. Heterogeneous *Helicobacter pylori* isolates from members of a family with a history of peptic ulcer disease. Gastroenterology 111:638-647.

[32] Vincent, P., F. Gottrand, P. Pernes, M. O. Husson, M. Lecomtehoucke, D. Turck, and H. Leclerc. 1994. High prevalence of Helicobacter pylori infection in cohabiting children—epidemiology of a cluster, with special emphasis on molecular typing. Gut 35:313-316.

[33] Rowland, M., L. Daly, M. Vaughan, A. Higgins, B. Bourke, and B. Drumm. 2006. Age-specific incidence of Helicobacter pylori. Gastroenterology 130: 65-72.

[34] Queralt, N., R. Bartolome, and R. Araujo. 2005. Detection of *Helicobacter*

pylori DNA in human faeces and water with different levels of faecal pollution in the north-east of Spain. J. Appl. Microbiol. 98:889-895.

[35] Laporte, R., P. Pernes, P. Pronnier, F. Gottrand, and P. Vincent. 2004. Acquisition of *Helicobacter pylori* infection after outbreaks of gastroenteritis: prospective cohort survey in institutionalised young people. BMJ 329: 204-205.

[36] Poms, R. E., and S. R. Tatini. 2001. Survival of Helicobacter pylori in ready-to-eat foods at 4 degrees C. Int. J. Food Microbiol. 63:281-286.

[37] Kusters, J. G., M. M. Gerrits, J. A. Van Strijp, and C. M. Vandenbroucke-Grauls. 1997. Coccoid forms of *Helicobacter pylori* are the morphologic manifestation of cell death. Infect. Immun. 65:3672-3679.

[38] Forman D., 1991, The etiology of gastric cancer. *fARC Sci. Publ. 105:22-32.*

[39] Hansson L. E., 2000, Risk of stomach cancer in patients with peptic ulcer disease. *World Surg.* 24(3):315-320.

[40] EI-Omar E. M., Oien K., Murray L. S., *et al.,* 2000, Increased prevalence of precancerous changes in relatives of gastric cancer patients: critical role of *H. pylori. Gastroenterology. 118(1):22-30.*

[41] Kuipers, E. J., J. C. Thijs, and H. P. Festen. 1995. The prevalence *of Helicobacter pylori* in peptic ulcer disease. Aliment. Pharmacol. Ther. 9(Suppl. 2):59-69.

[42] Kusters, J. G., Van Vliet, A. H., & Kuipers, E. J. (2006). Pathogenesis of *Helicobacter pylori* infection. *Clinical microbiology reviews*, *19*(3), 449-490.

[43] Sobala, G. M., J. E. Crabtree, M. F. Dixon, C. J. Schorah, J. D. Taylor, B. J. Rathbone, R. V. Heatley, and A. T. R. Axon. 1991. Acute *Helicobacter pylori* infection: clinical features, local and systemic immune response, gastric mucosal histology, and gastric juice ascorbic acid concentrations. Gut 32:1415-1418.

[44] Graham, D. Y., A. R. Opekun, M. S. Osato, H. M. El-Zimaity, C. K. Lee, Y. Yamaoka, W. A. Qureshi, M. Cadoz, and T. P. Monath. 2004. Challenge model for *Helicobacter pylori* infection in human volunteers. Gut 53:1235– 1243.

[45] Perez-Perez, G. I., R. B. Sack, R. Reid, M. Santosham, J. Croll, and M. J. Blaser. 2003. Transient and persistent *Helicobacter pylori* colonization in Native American children. J. Clin. Microbiol. 41:2401-2407.

[46] Malaty, H. M., L. Engstrand, N. L. Pedersen, and D. Y. Graham. 1994. *Helicobacter pylori* infection: genetic and environmental influences. A study of twins. Ann. Intern. Med. 120:982-986.

[47] Kuipers, E. J., A. M. Uyterlinde, A. S. Pena, H. J. Hazenberg, E. Bloemena, J. Lindeman, E. C. Klinkenberg-Knol, and S. G. Meuwissen. 1995. Increase of *Helicobacter pylori*-associated corpus gastritis during acid suppressive therapy: implications for long-term safety. Am. J. Gastroenterol. 90:1401– 1406.

[48] Ruiz, B., P. Correa, E. T. H. Fontham, and T. Ramakrishnan. 1996. Antral atrophy, Helicobacter pylori colonization, and gastric pH. Am. J. Clin. Pathol. 105:96-101

[49] Verdu', E., D. Armstrong, R. Fraser, F. Viani, J.-P. Idströ m, C. Cederberg, and A. L. Blum. 1995. Effect of *H. pylori* status on intragastric pH during treatment with omeprazole. Gut 36:539-543.

[50] Holtmann, G., C. Cain, and P. Malfertheiner. 1999. Gastric *Helicobacter pylori* infection accelerates healing of reflux esophagitis during treatment

with the proton pump inhibitor pantoprazole. Gastroenterology 117:11-16.

[51] El-Omar, E. M., M. Carrington, W. H. Chow, K. E. McColl, J. H. Bream, H. A. Young, J. Herrera, J. Lissowska, C. C. Yuan, N. Rothman, G. Lanyon, M. Martin, J. F. Fraumeni, Jr., and C. S. Rabkin. 2000. Interleukin-1 polymorphisms associated with increased risk of gastric cancer. Nature 404:398-402.

[52] Blaser, M. J., and J. C. Atherton. 2004. *Helicobacter pylori* persistence: biology and disease. J. Clin. Investig. 113:321-333.

[53] Leunk, R. D., P. T. Johnson, B. C. David, W. G. Kraft, and D. R. Morgan. 1988. Cytotoxic activity in broth-culture filtrates of *Campylobacter pylori*. J. Med. Microbiol. 26:93-99.

[54] Covacci, A., S. Censini, M. Bugnoli, R. Petracca, D. Burroni, G. Macchia, A. Massone, E. Papini, Z. Xiang, N. Figura, and R. Rappuoli. 1993. Molecular characterization of the 128-kDa immunodominant antigen of *Helicobacter pylori* associated with cytotoxicity and duodenal ulcer. Proc. Natl. Acad. Sci. USA 90:5791-5795.

[55] Tummuru, M. K. R., T. L. Cover, and M. J. Blaser. 1993. Cloning and expression of a high molecular mass major antigen of *Helicobacter pylori:* evidence of linkage to cytotoxin production. Infect. Immun. 61:1799-1809.

[56] van Doorn, L. J., C. Figueiredo, R. Sanna, M. J. Blaser, and W. G. Quint. 1999. Distinct variants of *Helicobacter pylori cagA* are associated with *vacA* subtypes. J. Clin. Microbiol. 37:2306-2311.

[57] Peek, R. M., G. G. Miller, K. T. Tham, G. I. Pe´rez-Pe´rez, X. M. Zhao, J. C. Atherton, and M. J. Blaser. 1995. Heightened inflammatory response and cytokine expression *in vivo* to *cagA_ Helicobacter pylori* strains. Lab. Investig. 73:760-770.

[58] Segal, E. D., J. Cha, J. Lo, S. Falkow, and L. S. Tompkins. 1999. Altered states: involvement of phosphorylated CagA in the induction of host cellular growth changes by *Helicobacter pylori*. Proc. Natl. Acad. Sci. USA. 96:14559-14564.

[59] Stein, M., R. Rappuoli, and A. Covacci. 2000. Tyrosine phosphorylation of the *Helicobacter pylori* CagA antigen after *cag*-driven host cell translocation. Proc. Natl. Acad. Sci. USA 97:1263-1268

[60] Stein, M., F. Bagnoli, R. Halenbeck, R. Rappuoli, W. J. Fantl, and A. Covacci. 2002. c-Src/Lyn kinases activate Helicobacter pylori CagA through tyrosine phosphorylation of the EPIYA motifs. Mol. Microbiol. 43:971-980.

[61] Selbach, M., S. Moese, S. Backert, P. R. Jungblut, and T. F. Meyer. 2004. The *Helicobacter pylori* CagA protein induces tyrosine dephosphorylation of ezrin. Proteomics 4:2961-2968.

[62] Smith, M. A., and D. I. Edwards. 1995. The influence of microaerophilia and anaerobiosis on metronidazole uptake in *Helicobacter pylori*. J. Antimicrob. Chemother. 36:453-461.

[63] Fischer, W., J. Puls, R. Buhrdorf, B. Gebert, S. Odenbreit, and R. Haas. 2001. Systematic mutagenesis of the *Helicobacter pylori* cag pathogenicity island: essential genes for CagA translocation in host cells and induction of interleukin-8. Mol. Microbiol. 42:1337-1348.

[64] Viala, J., C. Chaput, I. G. Boneca, A. Cardona, S. E. Girardin, A. P. Moran, R. Athman, S. Memet, M. R. Huerre, A. J. Coyle, P. S. DiStefano, P. J. Sansonetti, A. Labigne, J. Bertin, D. J. Philpott, and R. L. Ferrero. 2004. Nod1 responds to

peptidoglycan delivered by the *Helicobacter pylori* cag pathogenicity island. Nat. Immunol. 5:1166-1174.

[65] Tsutsumi, R., H. Higashi, M. Higuchi, M. Okada, and M. Hatakeyama. 2003. Attenuation of *Helicobacter pylori* CagA SHP-2 signaling by interaction between CagA and C-terminal Src kinase. J. Biol. Chem. 278:3664-3670.

[66] Higashi, H., R. Tsutsumi, A. Fujita, S. Yamazaki, M. Asaka, T. Azuma, and M. Hatakeyama. 2002. Biological activity of the *Helicobacter pylori* virulence factor CagA is determined by variation in the tyrosine phosphorylation sites. Proc. Natl. Acad. Sci. USA 99:14428-14433.

[67] Yamazaki, S., A. Yamakawa, Y. Ito, M. Ohtani, H. Higashi, M. Hatakeyama, and T. Azuma. 2003. The CagA protein of *Helicobacter pylori* is translocated into epithelial cells and binds to SHP-2 in human gastric mucosa. J. Infect. Dis. 187:334-337.

[68] Salama, N. R., G. Otto, L. Tompkins, and S. Falkow. 2001. Vacuolating cytotoxin of *Helicobacter pylori* plays a role during colonization in a mouse model of infection. Infect. Immun. 69:730-736

[69] van Doorn, L. J., C. Figueiredo, R. Sanna, S. Pena, P. Midolo, E. K. Ng, J. C. Atherton, M. J. Blaser, and W. G. Quint. 1998. Expanding allelic diversity of *Helicobacter pylori vacA*. J. Clin. Microbiol. 36:2597-2603.

[70] Montecucco, C., and M. de Bernard. 2003. Molecular and cellular mechanisms of action of the vacuolating cytotoxin (VacA) and neutrophil-activating protein (HP NAP) virulence factors of *Helicobacter pylori*. Microbes Infect. 5:715-721.

[71] Fitchen, N., D. P. Letley, P. O'Shea, J. C. Atherton, P. Williams, and K. R. Hardie. 2005. All subtypes of the cytotoxin VacA adsorb to the surface of *Helicobacter pylori* post-secretion. J. Med. Microbiol. 54:621-630.

[72] Torres, V. J., S. E. Ivie, M. S. McClain, and T. L. Cover. 2005. Functional properties of the p33 and p55 domains of the *Helicobacter pylori* vacuolating cytotoxin. J. Biol. Chem. 280:21107-21114.

[73] Telford, J. L., P. Ghiara, M. Dell'Orco, M. Comanducci, D. Burroni, M. Bugnoli, M. F. Tecce, S. Censini, A. Covacci, Z. Xiang, et al. 1994. Gene structure of the *Helicobacter pylori* cytotoxin and evidence of its key role in gastric disease. J. Exp. Med. 179:1653-1658.

[74] Pelicic, V., J. M. Reyrat, L. Sartori, C. Pagliaccia, R. Rappuoli, J. L. Telford, C. Montecucco, and E. Papini. 1999. *Helicobacter pylori* VacA cytotoxin associated with the bacteria increases epithelial permeability independently of its vacuolating activity. Microbiology 145:2043-2050

[75] Willhite, D. C., and S. R. Blanke. 2004. *Helicobacter pylori* vacuolating cytotoxin enters cells, localizes to the mitochondria, and induces mitochondrial membrane permeability changes correlated to toxin channel activity. Cell. Microbiol. 6:143-154.

[76] Neu, B., P. Randlkofer, M. Neuhofer, P. Voland, A. Mayerhofer, M. Gerhard, W. Schepp, and C. Prinz. 2002. *Helicobacter pylori* induces apoptosis of rat gastric parietal cells. Am. J. Physiol. Gastrointest. Liver Physiol. 283:G309–G318.

[77] Testerman, T. L., McGee, D. J., & Mobley, H. L. (2001). Adherence and colonization. *Helicobacter pylori: physiology and genetics*, 379-417.

[78] Logan R. P. H., 1996, Adherence of *Helicobacter pylori*. *Aliment Pharmacal. Ther.* 10(Supp!. I): 3-15.

[79] Dunn B. E., Altmann M., and Campbell G. P., 1991, Adherence of *Helicobacter pylori* to gastric carcinoma cells: Analysis by flow cytometry. *Rev. lrifect. Dis.* 13(Supp!. 8):S657-S664.

[80] Yamamoto-Osaki T, Yamaguchi H., Taguchi H., Ogata S., and Kamiya S., 1995, Adherence of *Helicabacter pylori* to cultured human gastric carcinoma cells. *Ear. J Gastroenterol. Hepatol.* 7(Supp!.I): S89-S92.

[81] Cole S. P., Cirillo D., Kagnoff M. F., Guiney O. G., and Eckmann L., 1997, Coccoid and spiral *Helicobacter pylori* differ in their abilities to adhere to gastric epithelial cells and induce interleukin-8 secretion. *lrifect. Immun. 65:843-·846.*

[82] Teyssen S, Chari ST, Scheid J, Singer MV. Effect of repeated boluses of intravenous omeprazole and primed infusions of ranitidine on 24-hour intragastric pH in healthy human subjects. Dig Dis Sci. 1995;40:247-55.

[83] Code CF. Defense mechanisms of the gastric mucosa. Scand J Gastroenterol Suppl. 1981;67:201-4.

[84] Henriksnas J, Phillipson M, Storm M, Engstrand L, Soleimani M, Holm L. Impaired mucus-bicarbonate barrier in *Helicobacter pylori* -infected mice. Am J Physiol Gastrointest Liver Physiol. 2006;291:G396-403.

[85] Baumgartner HK, Montrose MH. Regulated alkali secretion acts in tandem with unstirred layers to regulate mouse gastric surface pH. Gastroenterology. 2004;126:774-83.

[86] McGowan CC, Necheva AS, Forsyth MH, Cover TL, Blaser MJ. Promoter analysis of *Helicobacter pylori* genes with enhanced expression at low pH. Mol Microbiol. 2003;48:1225-39.

[87] Merrell DS, Goodrich ML, Otto G, Tompkins LS, Falkow S. pH-regulated gene expression of the gastric pathogen *Helicobacter pylori*. Infect Immun. 2003;71:3529-39.

[88] Wen Y, Marcus EA, Matrubutham U, Gleeson MA, Scott DR, Sachs G. Acid-adaptive genes of *Helicobacter pylori*. Infect Immun. 2003;71:5921-39.

[89] Larkin CJ, Watson RGP, Sloan JM, Stevenson M, Ardill JE, Buchanan D. Distribution of atrophy in *Helicobacter pylori* -infected subjects taking proton pump inhibitors. Scand J Gastroenterol. 2000;35:578-82.

[90] Lee A, Dixon MF, Danon SJ, Kuipers E, Megraud F, Larsson H, et al. Local acid production and *Helicobacter pylori*: a unifying hypothesis of gastroduodenal disease. Eur J Gastroenterol Hepatol. 1995;7:461-5.

[91] Logan RP, Walker MM, Misiewicz JJ, Gummett PA, Karim QN, Baron JH. Changes in the intragastric distribution of *Helicobacter pylori* during treatment with omeprazole. Gut. 1995;36:12-6.

[92] Mollenhauer-Rektorschek M, Hanauer G, Sachs G, Melchers K. Expression of UreI is required for intragastric transit and colonization of gerbil gastric mucosa by *Helicobacter pylori*. Res Microbiol. 2002;153:659-66.

[93] Scott DR, Marcus EA, Wen Y, Oh J, Sachs G. Gene expression *in vivo* shows that *Helicobacter pylori* colonizes an acidic niche on the gastric surface. Proc Natl Acad Sci U S A. 2007;104:7235-40.

[94] Hirayama F, Takagi S, Kusuhara H, Iwao E, Yokoyama Y, Ikeda Y. Induction of gastric ulcer and intestinal metaplasia in mongolian gerbils infected with *Helicobacter pylori*. J Gastroenterol. 1996;31: 755-7.

[95] Matsumoto S, Washizuka Y, Matsumoto Y, Tawara S, Ikeda F, Yokota Y, et al. Induction of ulceration

and severe gastritis in Mongolian gerbil by *Helicobacter pylori* infection. J Med Microbiol. 1997;46:391-7.

[96] Watanabe T, Tada M, Nagai H, Sasaki S, Nakao M. *Helicobacter pylori* infection induces gastric cancer in mongolian gerbils. Gastroenterology. 1998;115: 642-8.

[97] Dytoc M., Gold B., Louie M., et aI., 1993, Comparison of *Helicobacter pylori* and attaching effacing Escherichia coli adhesion to eukaryotic cells. lrifect. Immun. 61:448-456.

[98] O'Toole P. W, Janzon L., Doig P., Huang., Kostrzynska M., and Trust T., 1995, The putative neuraminyllactose-binding hemagglutinin HpaA of *Helicabacter pylori* CCUG 17874 is a lipoprotein. *J Bacterial.* 177:6049-605 7.

[99] Lingwood C. A, Huesca M., and Kuksis A, 1992, The glycerolipid receptor for *Helicobacter pylori* (and exoenzyme S) is phosphatidyiethanolamine. *lrifect. Immun. 60:2470-2474.*

[100] Boren T, Falk P., Roth K. A., Larson G., and Normark S., 1993, Attachment of *Helicobacter pylori* to human gastric epithelium mediated by blood group antigens. *Science 262: 1892-1895.*

[101] Kondo I., Nagate T., Akashi T., Kaneda Y, Miyachi J., and Yamaguchi M., 1993, Presence of receptors for laminin, collagen, fibronectin and vitronectin on the cell surface of *Helicobacter pylori*. *Eur.* J *Gastroentero!. Hepatol.* 5:S63-S67.

[102] Yamaguchi H., Osaki T., Kurihara N., *et aI.,* 1999, Induction of secretion of interleukin-8 from human gastric epithelial cells by heat-shock protein 60 homologue of *Helieobaeter pylori*. J *Med. Microbiol. 48:927-933.*

[103] Uibo R., Vorobjova T, Metskula K., Kisand K., Wadstrom T, and Kivik T, 1995, Association of *Helicohacter pylori* and gastric autoimmunity: a population based study, *FEMS Immunol. Med. Microbiol.* 11:65.

[104] Negrini R., Lisato L., Zanella 1., Cavazzini L., Gullini S., Vilianacci v., Poiesi C., Albertini A., and Ghielmi S., 1991, *Helicobacter pylori* infection induces antibodies cross-reacting with human gastric mucosa, *Gastroenterology 101:437.*

[105] Faller G., Steininger H., Kranzlein., Maul H., Kerkau T, Hensen., Hahn E. G., and Kirchner T, 1997, Antigastric autoantibodies in *Helicobacter pylori* infection: implications of histological and clinical parameters of gastritis, *Gut 41:619.*

[106] Schreiber S, Konradt M, Groll C, Scheid P, Hanauer G, Werling HO, et al. The spatial orientation of *Helicobacter pylori* in the gastric mucus. Proc Natl Acad Sci U S A. 2004;101:5024-9.

[107] Cerda O, Rivas A, Toledo H. *Helicobacter pylori* strain ATCC700392 encodes a methyl-accepting chemotaxis receptor protein (MCP) for arginine and sodium bicarbonate. FEMS Microbiol Lett. 2003; 224:175-81.

[108] Foynes S, Dorrell N, Ward SJ, Stabler RA, McColm AA, Rycroft AN, et al. *Helicobacter pylori* possesses two CheY response regulators and a histidine kinase sensor, CheA, which are essential for chemotaxis and colonization of the gastric mucosa. Infect Immun. 2000;68:2016-23.

[109] Nakamura H, Yoshiyama H, Takeuchi H, Mizote T, Okita K, Nakazawa T. Urease plays an important role in the chemotactic motility of *Helicobacter pylori* in a viscous environment. Infect Immun. 1998;66:4832-7.

[110] Sanders L, Andermann TM, Ottemann KM. A supplemented soft agar chemotaxis assay demonstrates the

Helicobacter pylori chemotactic response to zinc and nickel. Microbiology. 2013;159(Pt 1):46-57.

[111] Worku ML, Karim QN, Spencer J, Sidebotham RL. Chemotactic response of *Helicobacter pylori* to human plasma and bile. J Med Microbiol. 2004;53(Pt 8):807-11.

[112] Rader BA, Wreden C, Hicks KG, Sweeney EG, Ottemann KM, Guillemin K. *Helicobacter pylori* perceives the quorum-sensing molecule AI-2 as a chemorepellent via the chemoreceptor TlpB. Microbiology. 2011;157(Pt 9):2445-55.

[113] Schweinitzer T, Mizote T, Ishikawa N, Dudnik A, Inatsu S, Schreiber S, et al. Functional characterization and mutagenesis of the proposed behavioral sensor TlpD of *Helicobacter pylori*. J Bacteriol. 2008;190:3244-55.

[114] Boren T, Falk P, Roth KA, Larson G, Normark S. Attachment of *Helicobacter pylori* to human gastric epithelium mediated by blood group antigens. Science. 1993;262:1892-5.

[115] Sakamoto S, Watanabe T, Tokumaru T, Takagi H, Nakazato H, Lloyd KO. Expression of Lewisa, Lewisb, Lewisx, Lewisy, siayl-Lewisa, and sialyl- Lewisx blood group antigens in human gastric carcinoma and in normal gastric tissue. Cancer Res. 1989;49:745-52.

[116] Gerhard M, Lehn N, Neumayer N, Boren T, Rad R, Schepp W, et al. Clinical relevance of the *Helicobacter pylori* gene for blood-group antigen-binding adhesin. Proc Natl Acad Sci U S A. 1999; 96:12778-83.

[117] Ilver D, Arnqvist A, Ogren J, Frick IM, Kersulyte D, Incecik ET, et al. *Helicobacter pylori* adhesin binding fucosylated histo-blood group antigens revealed by retagging. Science. 1998; 279:373-7.

[118] Mahdavi J, Sonden B, Hurtig M, Olfat FO, Forsberg L, Roche N, et al. *Helicobacter pylori* SabA adhesion in persistent infection and chronic inflammation. Science. 2002;297:573-8.

[119] Ota H, Nakayama J, Momose M, Hayama M, Akamatsu T, Katsuyama T, et al. *Helicobacter pylori* infection produces reversible glycosylation changes to gastric mucins. Virchows Arch. 1998;433:419-26.

[120] Peck B, Ortkamp M, Diehl KD, Hundt E, Knapp B. Conservation, localization and expression of HopZ, a protein involved in adhesion of *Helicobacter pylori*. Nucleic Acids Res. 1999;27:3325-33.

[121] Odenbreit S, Faller G, Haas R. Role of the alpAB proteins and lipopolysaccharide in adhesion of *Helicobacter pylori* to human gastric tissue. Int J Med Microbiol. 2002;292:247-56.

[122] Marcus EA, Moshfegh AP, Sachs G, Scott DR. The periplasmic alpha-carbonic anhydrase activity of *Helicobacter pylori* is essential for acid acclimation. J Bacteriol. 2005;187:729-38.

[123] Ma Z, Gong S, Richard H, Tucker DL, Conway T, Foster JW. GadE (YhiE) activates glutamate decarboxylase- dependent acid resistance in *Escherichia coli* K-12. Mol Microbiol. 2003;49:1309-20.

[124] Booth IR. Regulation of cytoplasmic pH in bacteria. Microbiolo Rev. 1985;49:359-78.

[125] Padan E, Zilberstein D, Schuldiner S. pH homeostasis in bacteria. Biochim Biophys Acta. 1981;650:151-66.

[126] Tomb JF, White O, Kerlavage AR, Clayton RA, Sutton GG, Fleischmann RD, *et al.* The complete genome sequence of the gastric

pathogen *Helicobacter pylori*. Nature. 1997;388:539-47.

[127] Akada JK, Shirai M, Takeuchi H, Tsuda M, Nakazawa T. Identifi cation of the urease operon in *Helicobacter pylori* and its control by mRNA decay in response to pH. Mol Microbiol. 2000;36: 1071-84.

[128] Eaton KA, Brooks CL, Morgan DR, Krakowka S. Essential role of urease in pathogenesis of gastritis induced by *Helicobacter pylori* in gnotobiotic piglets. Infect Immun. 1991;59:2470-5.

[129] Eaton KA, Krakowka S. Effect of gastric pH on ureasedependent colonization of gnotobiotic piglets by *Helicobacter pylori*. Infect Immun. 1994;62:3604-7.

[130] Hu LT, Mobley HL. Purifi cation and N-terminal analysis of urease from *Helicobacter pylori*. Infect Immun. 1990; 58:992-8.

[131] Mobley HL, Hu LT, Foxal PA. *Helicobacter pylori* urease: properties and role in pathogenesis. Scand J Gastroenterol Suppl. 1991;187:39-46.

[132] Scott DR, Marcus EA, Weeks DL, Lee A, Melchers K, Sachs G. Expression of the *Helicobacter pylori ureI* gene is required for acidic pH activation of cytoplasmic urease. Infect Immun. 2000;68:470-7.

[133] Weeks DL, Eskandari S, Scott DR, Sachs G. A H+-gated urea channel: the link between *Helicobacter pylori* urease and gastric colonization. Science. 2000; 287:482-5.

[134] Ha NC, Oh ST, Sung JY, Cha KA, Lee MH, Oh BH. Supramolecular assembly and acid resistance of *Helicobacter pylori* urease. Nat Struct Biol. 2001;8:505-9.

[135] Scott DR, Marcus EA, Weeks DL, Sachs G. Mechanisms of acid resistance due to the urease system of *Helicobacter pylori*. Gastroenterology. 2002;123: 187-95.

[136] Ferrero RL, Cussac V, Courcoux P, Labigne A. Construction of isogenic urease-negative mutants of *Helicobacter pylori* by allelic exchange. J Bacteriol. 1992;174:4212-7.

[137] Heimer SR, Mobley HL. Interaction of *Proteus mirabilis* urease apoenzyme and accessory proteins identified with yeast two-hybrid technology. J Bacteriol. 2001;183:1423-33.

[138] Voland P, Weeks DL, Marcus EA, Prinz C, Sachs G, Scott D. Interactions among the seven *Helicobacter pylori* proteins encoded by the urease gene cluster. Am J Physiol Gastrointest Liver Physiol. 2003;284:G96-106.

[139] Moncrief MB, Hausinger RP. Purifi cation and activation properties of UreD-UreF-urease apoprotein complexes. J Bacteriol. 1996;178:5417-21.

[140] Moncrief MB, Hausinger RP. Characterization of UreG, identifi cation of a UreD-UreF-UreG complex, and evidence suggesting that a nucleotide-binding site in UreG is required for *in vivo* metallocenter assembly of *Klebsiella aerogenes* urease. J Bacteriol. 1997;179: 4081-6.

[141] Park IS, Carr MB, Hausinger RP. In vitro activation of urease apoprotein and role of UreD as a chaperone required for nickel metallocenter assembly. Proc Natl Acad Sci U S A. 1994;91:3233-7.

[142] van Vliet AH, Ernst FD, Kusters JG. NikR-mediated regulation of *Helicobacter pylori* acid adaptation. Trends Microbiol. 2004;12:489-94.

[143] Carpenter BM, West AL, Gancz H, Servetas SL, Pich OQ, Gilbreath JJ, et al. Crosstalk between the *Hp* ArsRS

two-component system and *Hp* NikR is necessary for maximal activation of urease transcription. Front Microbiol. 2015;6:558.

[144] Dosanjh NS, Hammerbacher NA, Michel SL. Characterization of the *Helicobacter pylori* NikR-*P* (*ureA*) DNA interaction: metal ion requirements and sequence specifi city. Biochemistry. 2007;46:2520-9.

[145] Dosanjh NS, West AL, Michel SL. *Helicobacter pylori* NikR's interaction with DNA: a two-tiered mode of recognition. Biochemistry. 2009;48:527-36.

[146] Evans SE, Michel SL. Dissecting the role of DNA sequence in *Helicobacter pylori* NikR/DNA recognition. Dalton Trans. 2012;41:7946-51.

[147] Mohammadi, M., S. Czinn, R. Redline, and J. Nedrud. 1996. Helicobacter specific cell-mediated immune responses display a pre-dominant Th1 phenotype and promote a delayed-type hypersensitivity response in the stomachs of mice. J. Immunol. 156:4729-4738

[148] Sommer, F., H. Wilken, G. Faller, and M. Lohoff. 2004. Systemic Th1 immunization of mice against *Helicobacter pylori* infection with CpG oligodeoxynucleotides as adjuvants does not protect from infection but enhances gastritis. Infect. Immun. 72:1029-1035

Chapter 7

Gastrointestinal Physiopathological Testing for Upper GI Functional Disorders

Edda Battaglia, Maria Luisa Niola, Valentina Boano, Chiara M.C. Elia, Carlo Sguazzini and Mario Grassini

Abstract

Functional gastrointestinal disorders (FGIDs) are disorders of gut–brain interaction; it is a group of disorders classified by gastrointestinal (GI) symptoms related to any combination of the following: motility disturbance, visceral hypersensitivity, altered mucosal and immune function, altered gut microbiota, altered central nervous system processing. In general, investigations on intestinal motility should be reserved for patients with symptoms correlated to motor alterations that greatly influence the quality of life, nutrition and productivity, as they are justified only if a result can be expected that influences the clinical management of the patient. Esophageal High-resolution manometry (HRM) today permits greater understanding of the function of the esophagogastric junction and the esophageal motility. In the more frequent clinical manifestation, like as Gastroesophageal reflux disease (GERD), despite endoscopy, the pH-impedance is considered the most accurate and detailed method to assess acid/weakly acid or non acid gastroesophageal reflux, to identify the specific phenotypes of reflux disease spectrum. To investigate gastric motor function, the scintigraphic gastric emptying test is the gold standard, but it still has poor uniformity of the protocols, that undermine the quality and usefulness of the test. The current and increasingly widespread alternative to scintigraphic emptying is the breath-test with octanoic acid (OBT) or Spirulina labeled with C13, a test that has the favor of not using radioactive substances and that has shown a high concordance with the scintigraphic test. The intraluminal capsule test is a recent promising tool, that records intraluminal pH, pressure, temperature and post-prandial gastric contractions, and transmits wireless data to a receiver. EGG is a non-invasive technique that measures gastric myoelectric activity- and consequently its function- using skin electrodes placed in the upper abdomen. Gastro-jejunal manometry with multiple pressure sensor catheters located in the antrum, pylorus, duodenum and jejunum is the only clinically available test that allows detailed evaluation of coordinated gastro-duodenum-jejunal contraction models. The functional ultrasound, the barostat, the SPECT and resonance methods have provided preliminary data on their application in the study of gastrointestinal motility, but the data are still missing and the methods are not validated.

Keywords: functional gastrointestinal disorders, functional tests, manometry, pH-impedance

IntechOpen

1. Introduction

Functional gastrointestinal disorders (FGIDs) are disorders of gut–brain interaction; it is a group of disorders classified by gastrointestinal (GI) symptoms related to any combination of the following: motility disturbance, visceral hypersensitivity, altered mucosal and immune function, altered gut microbiota, altered central nervous system processing [1].

2. Esophageal function

The evaluation of the esophageal function is not clearly defined because its dysfunction is mainly due to neuromuscular disorders, so its pathophysiology is complex.

However, esophageal manometry and 24-hour pH-impedance monitoring are two useful tests to classify the organ's disorders [2].

2.1 Manometry

Manometry is considered as the gold standard [3] to diagnose motor alterations of the esophagus. Conventional examination uses mostly water-perfused probes, with recording points placed every 5 cm along the length of the esophageal catheter, in order to measure internal contraction and pressure. However, high-resolution manometry (HRM) is nowadays the most accurate and available tool. HRM is equipped with high-resolution solid-state catheters that transmit data on the internal condition of the esophagus, which are then converted into graphs (topography plots, EPTs). The probes are placed every 1 cm, for a total of 32–36 transducers all along the organ [4].

In the standard procedure the patient is placed in a supine position in order to eliminate the gravitational effect, and a basal recording is made for 30 seconds, followed by at least 10 consecutive swallowings, during which various parameters of esophageal peristalsis are detected and recorded, the main ones being DCI (Distal Contractile Integral) and DL (Distal Latency).

The DCI represents the contractile vigor of the esophagus, i.e., amplitude x duration x length of contraction of the distal esophagus with an isobaric contour of 20 mmHg.

The DL (measured in seconds) is the interval between relaxation of the UES and the point of deflection along the 30 mmHg isobaric contour where the propulsion velocity slows (contractile deceleration point, CDP): it represents an indirect measure of post-deglutitive inhibition and thus normal peristalsis [3].

It has to be mentioned the IRP (Integrated Relaxation Pressure, in mmHg), which is defined as the mean pressure of the EGJ measured for 4 contiguous or not-relaxation seconds, during the ten seconds following deglutive relaxation of the UES [5].

The first step of the data analysis is focalized on the evaluation of the esophagogastric junction (EGJ): basal pressure of the lower esophageal sphincter (LES), IRP and crural diaphragm (CD) are evaluated, and junction subtypes are defined.

The Lyon Consensus [6] proposes to study EGJ in two different ways, from an anatomic and morphologic point of view and then from his contractility.

Morphologically, three types of junctions are described, where type 3 is associated with decreased LES pressure due to anatomical separation >3 cm between LES and CD. By the second measurement the EGJ-CI (EGJ Contractile Integral) is calculated, which measures the level of barrier provided by the junction.

The second step is about evaluating the peristalsis of the esophageal body, based on various parameters including the DCI and the interruptions of the isobaric contour of 20 mmHg, although with the latest Chicago classification (CC v3.0) it has been proposed to eliminate this last parameter from the assessment of esophageal contractile force, and to consider it as a descriptor of the contractile pattern [7]. So, contractile vigor can be described as absent (DCI <100 mmHg·s·cm), weak (DCI >100 but <450), inefficient (absent or weak), or hypercontractile (DCI ≥8000); contractile pattern instead can be premature (DL >4.5 sec), fragmented (interruptions >5 cm on the isobaric contour with DCI >450) or normal [3, 5].

Basing on the results obtained from the manometry, the patient is included in one of the four groups describing esophageal motility, as defined in CC v3.0 [8]:

- incomplete relaxation of the LES, such as achalasia subtypes I and III or EGJ outflow obstruction;
- major peristalsis disorders, such as distal esophageal spasm, esophageal 'jackhammer' hypercontractility, or absent contractility;
- minor motor disorders, such as fragmented peristalsis or ineffective esophageal motility (IEM);
- normal esophageal motility (**Figure 1**).

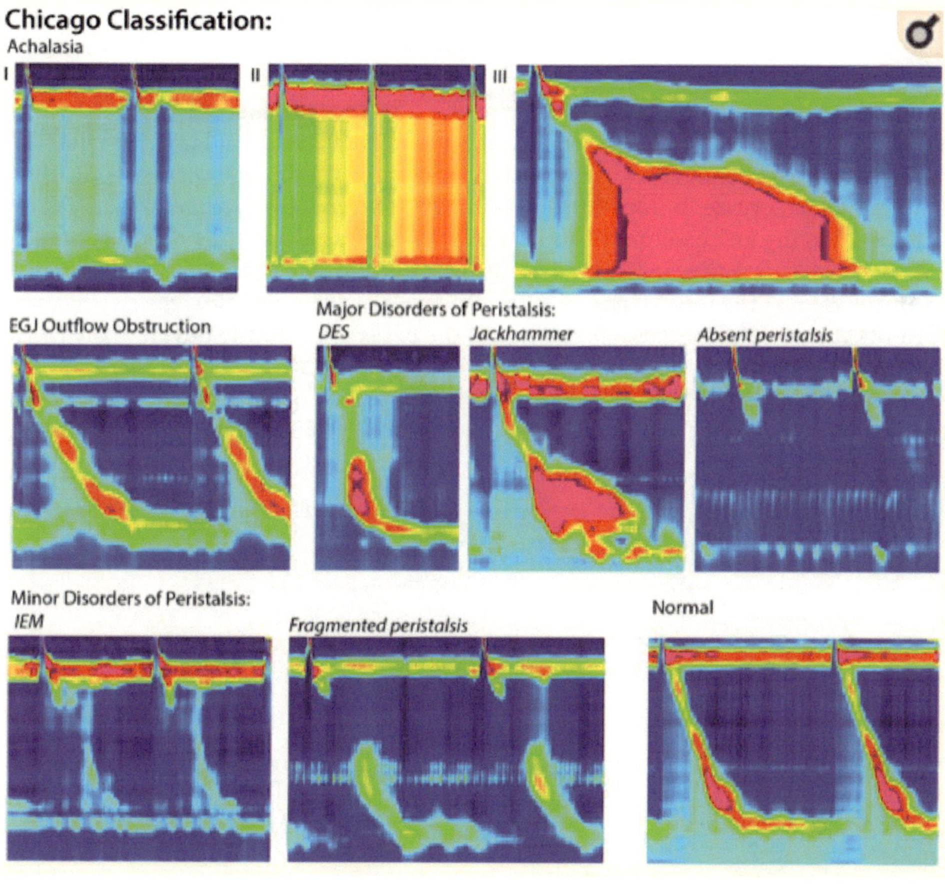

Figure 1.
Chicago classification on HRM [8].

2.2 24-hour pH-impedance monitoring

24-hour pH-impedance monitoring is today the most useful and sensitive test to study every type of reflux episode, its composition, proximal extension, duration and clearance. It is based on the simultaneous measurement of pH and endoluminal electrical impedance: a pair of electrodes correspond to an impedance segment that provides a measure of impedance (resistance): it is inversely proportional to conductivity, increasing if air is passing through the esophagus and decreasing if water/swallowed material or reflux is passing through it [9].

By combining the two measurement, the chemical nature and the physical nature of the reflux episode can be defined as acid, weakly acidic, weakly alkaline and liquid, gaseous or mixed.

Changes in pH occurred simultaneously with impedance drops of at least 50% are classified as follows:

- Acid reflux: a drop in pH <4 from a pre-event pH >4, lasting >5 seconds;
- Superimposed acid reflux: liquid reflux monitored by impedance electrodes while the esophageal pH is still <4, i.e., the pH in the distal esophagus has not returned to >4 after an episode of acid reflux;
- Weakly acid reflux: the pH nadir is ≥4 but <7 during reflux;
- Weakly alkaline reflux: no acid is present as the intra-esophageal pH increases to ≥7 or remains ≥7 during reflux (**Figure 2**).

Furthermore, a liquid episode is defined as a retrograde flux (to the proximal esophagus) capable of changing the basal impedance value by at least 50% in two consecutive channels; a gaseous episode, on the other hand, corresponds to a simultaneous increase in impedance >3000 Ω in two consecutive channels, with a channel having an absolute value >7000 Ω. Finally, a mixed episode is a gaseous reflux that occurs during or immediately after a liquid one [10].

By measuring the impedance on different levels of the esophagus the extension of reflux can be determined; it is relevant if the pH is altered at 15 cm cranially from the LES [11]. Moreover, the Acid Exposure Time (AET) can be calculated: a total exposure of less than 4% is judged normal while a value >6% is surely pathologic, and the total number of refluxes is considered normal if <54 [12]. The temporal

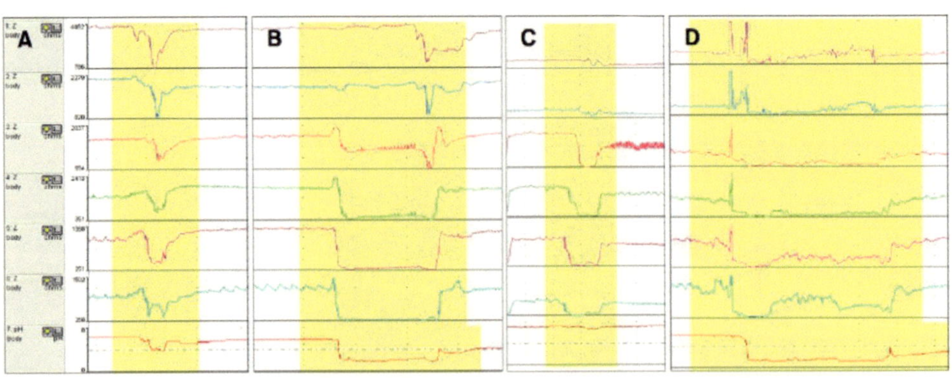

Figure 2.
(A) Weakly acidic reflux episode, (B) acidic episode, (C) weakly alkaline episode, (D) superimposed episode [9].

correlation between reflux episodes and symptoms is analyzed by measuring three parameters: the Symptom Index (SI), the Symptom Association Probability (SAP) and the Symptom Sensitivity Index (SSI). Additionally, two more parameters have been recently introduced, namely the Post reflux Swallow- induced Peristaltic Wave (PSPW) index, and the Mean Nocturnal Baseline Impedance (MNBI). The former refers to a vagal reflex that is activated after reflux and consists of swallowing that raises esophageal pH. The latter reflects the permeability of the esophageal mucosa and low values are related to alterations in tight junctions[1]. Thus, calculation of MNBI and PSPW together is useful in general to improve the yield of pH-impedance testing [13], and is particularly advantageous when the diagnosis of gastroesophageal reflux disease is doubtful (e.g., with normal AET and discordant SAP and SI) to distinguish patients with hypersensitive esophagus from patients with functional heartburn [14].

In conclusion, 24-hour pH-impedance monitoring is a test which is not so specific for functional disorders, but it allows to analyze multiple parameters. It allows therefore to make a diagnosis of gastroesophageal reflux disease, or to exclude it when there are doubts, as well as to distinguish the typical forms of reflux from those belonging to functional disorders (for example functional heartburn or reflux hypersensitivity).

3. Gastric function

The main tests to study the stomach function are gastric barostat, scintigraphy, tests using an intraluminal capsule, breath test, electrogastrography (EGG) and Water Load Test (WLT).

3.1 Barostat

Gastric barostat studies are the best-established methods of measuring gastric accommodation, and they are considered as the gold standard.

The barostat is a computerized air pump device that measures fundic relaxation in response to a meal, by monitoring the volume of air within an intragastric bag (a polyethylene balloon [15]) that is clamped at a constant pressure level [16]. The system maintains a constant pressure by fixing it and changes the bag's volume reflecting gastric relaxation or contraction (**Figure 3**). In this way, gastric accommodation response to various interventions is recorded.

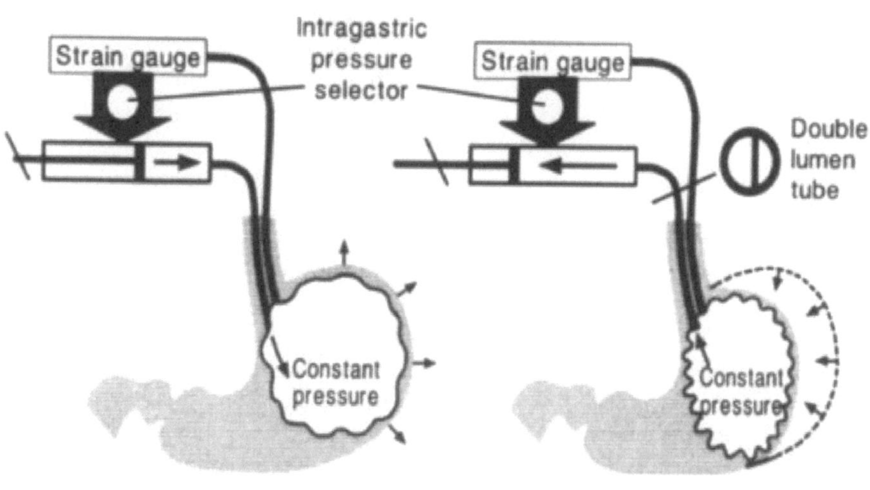

Figure 3.
Working mechanism of a barostat balloon [16].

The problem is that the barostat is an invasive test [17]: although it is a valuable technique, it is not practical in daily clinical assessment for patients nor for research studies. This is the reason why today non-invasive methods are preferred, and they will be later described in this chapter. Moreover, the barostat balloon can't perfectly measure post-prandial accommodation of the entire stomach, and it is possible that it interferes with the intra-gastric management of the meal [18] (**Figure 3**).

3.2 Scintigraphy

Gastric Emptying Scintigraphy (GES) is a non-invasive test that uses 99mTc-Nanocolloidal as the radioactive substance. The patient is usually given a solid and radiolabeled meal, then data are acquired, and the emptying time is analyzed. A liquid meal with water labeled with indium-111 diethylenetriaminopentacetic acid may also be used. The procedure should be repeated after 1 hour, 2 hours and 4 hours: in fact, delayed gastric emptying is detected with greater sensitivity at 4 hours, and images detect gastroparesis with 30% greater frequency. Imaging at 0,1,2 and 4 hours allows identification of both rapid and delayed gastric emptying, which is important because patients are treated in a different way, even though their symptoms are similar. Moreover, images at 60 minutes have a specificity and sensitivity of 90% for rapid gastric emptying, whereas images at 240 minutes show a specificity of 70% and sensitivity of 100% for delayed one [19]. Delayed emptying is considered to be gastric retention of more than 90% at 1 hour, more than 60% at 2 hours, and more than 10% at 4 hours [20].

3.3 Intraluminal capsule

The capsule test is performed by ingesting a capsule with the meal: this records intraluminal pH, pressure, temperature and post-prandial gastric contractions, and transmits wireless data to a receiver. In healthy people it is detected in the duodenum after about 5 hours. The test has a concordance of 90% with scintigraphic tests and has excellent sensitivity and specificity especially in detecting gastroparesis [21]. This technique offers a non-radioactive, ambulatory alternative to scintigraphy [22].

3.4 Breath test

A functional test for the study of gastric emptying (GE) is the breath test (GEBT) [23]. It is a non-invasive method, feasible also in pregnancy and children, that does not use any radiation, it is easily repeatable, and it is based on the measurement of the 13CO2/12CO2 ratio in the exhaled breath after the administration of a standard meal, labeled with 13C-Spirulina or 13C-Acetate or 13C-Octanoic Acid. The procedure is repeated at 45, 90, 120, 150, 180, and even 240 minutes after the end of the meal. By measuring the change in this ratio over time from the pre-meal value, the rate of 13CO2 excretion can be calculated and the individual's rate of gastric emptying determined.

When compared with scintigraphy, it showed similar values: good agreement was found between the two tests, thus validating the breath test as an alternative method for studying gastric emptying. Based on the study of normal values, the 10th and 90th percentiles of t 1/2 calculated with scintigraphy were used to classify patients as follows: subjects with delayed ($t1/2 > 86$ min), accelerated ($t1/2 < 52$ min), or normal (t1/2 52–86 min) [24] gastric emptying.

3.5 Electrogastrography (EGG)

EGG is a non-invasive technique that measures gastric myoelectric activity- and consequently its function- using skin electrodes placed in the upper abdomen. Normal activity consists of slow waves ad potential spikes (which would correspond to contractions), and the normal frequency is approximately 3 wpm [25].

The correlation between EGG and gastric emptying has been reported in several studies: in patients with functional dyspepsia, 40% of patients showed abnormal EGG [26]. The presence of EGG abnormalities in patients with dyspepsia or delayed gastric emptying, and the presence of motor abnormalities in many patients with GERD, leads to the conclusion that EGG abnormalities can be detected in some patients with gastroesophageal reflux disease, too.

3.6 Water Load Test

The Water Load Test is an economic, non-invasive and easy to perform test, that can be reproduced in healthy subjects as well as in patients with reflux disease or functional dyspepsia [27]. It is useful to assess visceral hypersensitivity, that has been identified as an important pathophysiologic mechanism in patients with functional disorders of the upper gastrointestinal tract [28].

The test consists of having the patient drink as much water as possible, consecutively for 5 minutes (WL5), or until a feeling of satiety is reached. The patients have to complete a visual analogue scale (VAS) in order to objectivate their symptoms before and after the test, and they have to assign a value for each of them, scaled from 0 (absent) to 10 (severe). Then, water is consumed from an unmasked flask that is refilled after each drink, but the patients are blinded as to the actual volume of water consumed. Finally, the total volume of water ingested, and the perceived symptoms are registered and analyzed [29].

There is also evidence that some GERD patients, more often with non-erosive disease, may improve dyspeptic symptoms after acid-suppression therapy [25]; however, large cohort studies suggest that that the reflux patients and dyspeptic patients represent two distinct populations [26]: GERD patients with mild erosive oesophagitis and with non-erosive reflux disease have the WLT abnormal, similar but not identical to that reported in patients with functional dyspepsia [29]. The WLT does not allow a precise determination of visceral hypersensitivity; however, it is worth noting that these findings appear somewhat similar to those described in other studies by means of the barostat technique in dyspeptic patients, although a correlation between these two methods is still not available. Although there is literature evidence suggesting abnormalities of gastric motor and sensory function in GERD patients [30, 31].

3.7 Other tests

Although these tests were not created exclusively to study gastric function, they are becoming a useful help in order to assess its accommodation in a non-invasive way: ultrasonography, magnetic resonance (MRI) and Single-proton Emission Computed Tomography (SPECT) are some examples.

Ultrasound imaging is a widely available method but offers only an indirect measure of gastric accommodation through antral diameter [17]. On the other hand, MRI is able to provide information about gastric meal emptying, the total volume of gastric contents and also three-dimensional images of the stomach [32].

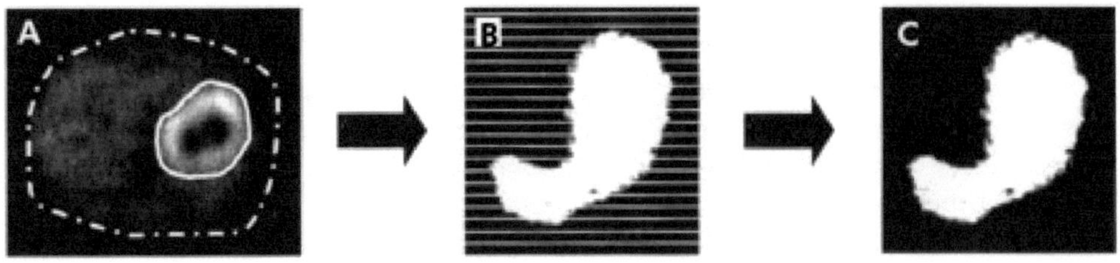

Figure 4.
(A) Multiple SPECT images are reconstructed with the help of a software system (B) into a three-dimensional image of the stomach (C) for the measurements of gastric volumes [35].

SPECT is an emerging test that uses intravenous injection of ^{99m}Tc-pertechnetate with tomographic imaging (three-dimensional reconstruction) of gastric mucosa. The evaluation of gastric accommodation is completed by measuring gastric volumes in fasting and post-prandial state [33] and by analyzing them with a commercially available software. Mean volumes detected by SPECT are comparable to that of barostat; moreover, it permits simultaneous assessment of gastric emptying and accommodation [34] (**Figure 4**).

4. Clinical usefulness

In what clinical conditions is it correct to perform these tests?

For standard esophageal manometry or HR esophageal manometry and reflux monitoring recent guidelines have given clear and shared indications [3, 4]. The utility of esophageal manometry in clinical practice is to accurately define esophageal motor function, to identify abnormal motor function, and to establish a treatment plan based on motor abnormalities, in patients with dysphagia, chest pain or in GERD patients before surgery.

Reflux testing has generally no indication in the majority of patients with typical GERD symptoms (i.e., heartburn and/or regurgitation) who have adequate symptom relief with medical therapy. The role of reflux monitoring is more important in patients with reflux symptoms and without endoscopic mucosal breaks, in whom an objective diagnostic test to define their disease is more likely to be needed. The prolonged reflux monitoring with pH-impedance catheter actually represents the most sensitive tool to document the role of reflux in patients with GERD symptoms. A further indication for reflux testing is represented by belching disorders and one of the most common use of reflux monitoring is the evaluation of patients with persistent typical GERD symptoms despite medical therapy, when refractory heartburn can be defined as the presence of heartburn that does not respond to at least 8-weeks of double-dose acid suppressing medications [4]. Furthermore it's recommended the evaluation of patients with esophageal symptoms suggestive for GERD before surgery, to confirm the reflux and the evaluation of children with symptoms suggestive for GERD (particularly in case of neurological symptoms and low growth).

As regards gastro-jejunal functional tests, there are no guidelines or consensus, but, extrapolating the data from the literature, we can consider these data useful in:

- Severe functional dyspepsia and related syndromes.
- Rumination symptoms.
- Atypical/estraesophagel forms of reflux.

- Pseudo-obstruction symptoms.

- Diabetes mellitus with functional symptoms and/or difficult metabolic compensation.

- Suspected gastroparesis (including post-surgery).

- Functional pre-intervention evaluation (plastic antireflux, colectomies for constipation, implantation of gastric pacemakers).

- Identification of specific feeding site enteral or for the administration of drugs enterally (Parkinson's).

5. Conclusions

The gastrointestinal functional tests represent the study modalities of esophageal-gastric motility and intestine, useful for the diagnostic definition and therapeutic management of functional gastric and intestinal disorders. These diseases affect a large proportion of the world population, compromise the quality of life and cause significant health care costs. It is important to underline that functional tests must always be preceded by a careful clinical evaluation that excludes other etiologies. In general, investigations on intestinal motility should be reserved for patients with symptoms correlated to motor alterations that greatly influence the quality of life, nutrition and productivity, as they are justified only if a result can be expected that influences the clinical management of the patient [36].

Author details

Edda Battaglia*, Maria Luisa Niola, Valentina Boano, Chiara M.C. Elia, Carlo Sguazzini and Mario Grassini
Physiopathology and Manometry Section, Gastroenterology and Endoscopy Unit, Cardinal Massaia Hospital, ASL AT, Asti, Italy

*Address all correspondence to: edda.battaglia@gmail.com

References

[1] Drossman DA. Functional gastrointestinal Disorders: History, Pathophysiology, Clinical Features, and Rome IV. Gastroenterology. 2016; 150:1262-79.

[2] Ang D, Fock KM, Law NM, Ang TL. Current status of functional gastrointestinal evaluation in clinical practice. Singapore Med J. 2015 Feb; 56(2):69-79; quiz 80. doi: 10.11622/smedj.2015021. Erratum in: Singapore Med J. 2015 Mar; 56(3):179.

[3] Savarino E, de Bortoli N, Bellini M, Galeazzi F, Ribolsi M, Salvador R et al. Practice guidelines on the use of esophageal manometry – A GISMAD-SIGE-AIGO medical position statement. Dig Liver Dis. 2016; 48(10):1124-35.

[4] Baldwin D, Puckett Y. Esophageal Manometry. [Updated 2020 Jun 14]. In: StatPearls [Internet]. Treasure Island (FL): StatPearls Publishing; 2020 Jan-. Available from: https://www.ncbi.nlm.nih.gov/books/NBK559237/

[5] Yadlapati R. High-resolution esophageal manometry: interpretation in clinical practice. Curr Opin Gastroenterol. 2017; 33(4):301-9.

[6] Gyawali CP, Kahrilas PJ, Savarino E, Zerbib F, Mion F, Smout A et al. Modern diagnosis of GERD: the Lyon Consensus. Gut. 2018; 67:1351-62.

[7] Kahrilas PJ, Bredenoord AJ, Fox M, Gyawali CP, Roman S, Smout AJ et al. The Chicago Classification of esophageal motility disorders, v3.0. Neurogastroenterol Motil. 2015; 27(2):160-74.

[8] Rohof WO, Bredenoord AJ. Chicago Classification of Esophageal Motility Disorders: Lessons Learned. Curr Gastroenterol Rep. 2017; 19(8):37.

[9] Cho YK. How to Interpret Esophageal Impedance pH Monitoring. J Neurogastroenterol Motil. 2010; 16(3):327-30.

[10] Savarino E, Frazzoni M, Marabotto E, Zentilin P, Iovino P, Costantini M et al. A SIGE- SINGEM-AIGO technical review on the clinical use of esophageal reflux monitoring. Dig Liver Dis. 2020; 52(9):966-80.

[11] Gyawali CP, Kahrilas PJ, Savarino E, Zerbib F, Mion F, Smout A et al. Modern diagnosis of GERD: the Lyon Consensus. Gut. 2018; 67:1351-62.

[12] Zentilin P, Iiritano E, Dulbecco P, Bilardi C, Savarino E, De Conca S et al. Normal values of 24-h ambulatory intraluminal impedance combined with pH-metry in subjects eating a Mediterranean diet. Dig Liver Dis. 2006; 38(4):226-32.

[13] Frazzoni M, Savarino E, de Bortoli N, Martinucci I, Furnari M, Frazzoni L et al. Analyses of the Post-reflux Swallow-induced Peristaltic Wave Index and Nocturnal Baseline Impedance Parameters Increase the Diagnostic Yield of Impedance-pH Monitoring of Patients with Reflux Disease. Clin Gastroenterol Hepatol. 2016; 14(1):40-46.

[14] Frazzoni M, de Bortoli N, Frazzoni L, Furnari M, Martinucci I, Tolone S et al. Impairment of chemical clearance and mucosal integrity distinguishes hypersensitive esophagus from functional heartburn. J Gastroenterol. 2017; 52(4):444-51.

[15] Amiriani T, Javadi H, Raiatnavaz T, Pashazadeh AM, Semnani S, Tabib SM, Assadi M. Assessment of Gastric Accommodation in Patients with Functional Dyspepsia by 99mTc-Pertechtenate Single Photon Emission Computed Tomography Imaging: Practical but not Widely Accepted. Mol Imaging Radionucl Ther. 2015 Oct 5;24(3):105-9.

[16] Azpiroz F, Malagelada JR. Gastric tone measured by an electronic barostat in health and postsurgical gastroparesis. Gastroenterology. 1987; 92:934-43.

[17] Schwizer W, Steingötter A, Fox M, et al. Non-invasive measurement of gastric accommodation in humans. Gut 2002;51: i59-i62.

[18] Kim DY, Camilleri M. Noninvasive measurement of gastric accommodation by SPECT. Korean J Intern Med. 2002 Mar; 17(1):1-6.

[19] Farrell MB. Gastric Emptying Scintigraphy. J Nucl Med Technol. 2019; 47(2):111-19;

[20] Abell TL, Camilleri M, Donohoe K, Hasler WL, Lin HC, Maurer AH et al. American Neurogastroenterology and Motility Society and the Society of Nuclear Medicine. Consensus recommendations for gastric emptying scintigraphy: a joint report of the American Neurogastroenterology and Motility Society and the Society of Nuclear Medicine. Am J Gastroenterol. 2008 Mar;103(3):753-63.

[21] Kuo B, McCallum RW, Koch KL, Sitrin MD, Wo JM, Chey WD et al. Comparison of gastric emptying of a nondigestible capsule to a radio-labelled meal in healthy and gastroparetic subjects. Aliment Pharmacol Ther. 2008;27(2):186-96.

[22] Saps M, Di Lorenzo C. 29 - Gastric Motility Disorders, In: Wyllie R, Hyams JS (editors). Pediatric Gastrointestinal and Liver Disease (Fourth Edition). WB Saunders. 2011; p. 309-318.e4.

[23] Bharucha AE, Camilleri M, Veil E, Burton D, Zinsmeister AR. Comprehensive assessment of gastric emptying with a stable isotope breath test. Neurogastroenterol Motil. 2013; 25(1): e60-e69.

[24] Szarka LA, Camilleri M, Vella A, Burton D, Baxter K, Simonson J et al. A stable isotope breath test with a standard meal for abnormal gastric emptying of solids in the clinic and in research. Clin Gastroenterol Hepatol. 2008; 6(6):635-43.e1.

[25] Yin J, Chen JD. Electrogastrography: methodology, validation and applications. J Neurogastroenterol Motil. 2013; 19(1):5-17.

[26] Chen CL, Hu CT, Lin HH, Yi CH. Clinical utility of electrogastrography and the water load test in patients with upper gastrointestinal symptoms. J Smooth Muscle Res. 2006; 42(5):149-57.

[27] Battaglia E, Grassini M, Navino M, Niola P, Verna C et al. Water load test before and after PPI therapy in patients with gastro-oesophageal reflux disease. Dig Liver Dis. 2007; 39(12):1052-56.

[28] Sarnelli G, Vandenberghe J, Tack J. Visceral hypersensitivity in functional disorders of the upper gastrointestinal tract. Dig Liver Dis. 2004; 36:371-6.

[29] Chen CL, Lin HH, Chen MC, Huang LC. Dyspeptic symptoms and water load test in patients with functional dyspepsia and reflux disease. Scand J Gastroenterol. 2005; 40(1):28-32.

[30] Parkman HP, Fisher RS. Contributing role of motility abnormalities in the pathogenesis of gastroesophageal reflux disease. Dig Dis 1997;15(Suppl. 1):40-52.

[31] Zerbib F, des Varannes SB, Ropert A, Lamouliatte H, Quinton A, Galmiche JP. Proximal gastric tone in gastro-oesophageal reflux disease. Eur J Gastroenterol Hepatol 1999;11:511-5.

[32] Schwizer W, Maecke H, Fried M. Measurement of gastric emptying by magnetic resonance imaging in humans. Gastroenterology. 1992;103(2):369-76.

[33] Kim DY, Camilleri M. Noninvasive measurement of gastric accommodation

by SPECT. Korean J Intern Med. 2002 Mar;17(1):1-6.

[34] Hong SP. Assessment of Gastric Accommodation by SPECT. J Neurogastroenterol Motil. 2010 Oct;16(4):347-9. Epub 2010 Oct 30.

[35] Bouras EP, Delgado-Aros S, Camilleri M et al. SPECT imaging of the stomach: comparison with barostat, and effects of sex, age, body mass index, and fundoplication. Gut 2002; 51:781-6.

[36] Battaglia E, Boano V, Sguazzini CE, Elia CM, Grassini M. Gastrointestinal physiopatological testing: what's new? Minerva Gastroenterol Dietol. 2020;6(1):1-3

Chapter 8

Gastroduodenal Lesions Associated with Portal Hypertension: An Extensive Review

Vincenzo Neri, Nicola Tartaglia, Alberto Fersini, Pasquale Cianci, Mario Pacilli, Giovanna Pavone and Antonio Ambrosi

Abstract

The block of the portal flow by obstacles in prehepatic, hepatic or posthepatic site and alterations of the splanchnic blood flow are the pathological conditions that lead to portal hypertension. The portal hypertension can cause also others gastroduodenal lesions, potentially hemorrhagic, in addition to esophageal varices commonly developed and habitual source of bleeding in these patients. The gastroduodenal lesions associated with portal hypertension, usually encountered in the clinical practice, are portal hypertensive gastropaty, gastric antral vascular ectasia, gastric and duodenal ulcer, isolated gastric varices. The pathophysiology and clinical, diagnostic and therapeutic features of these lesions are examined.

Keywords: portal hypertension, portal hypertensive gastropathy, gastric antral vascular ectasia, peptic ulcer bleeding, gastric varices

1. Introduction

Hepatic fibrosis, nodular rigeneration, distortion of hepatic architecture are the histopathological characters of liver cirrhosis. The main outcome of this pathological condition is the portal hypertension (PH) by the disruption of the hepatic blood flow, beside the damage of liver metabolic functions. Moreover the alteration of the splanchnic blood flow and the block of portal flow can be localized also in the prehepatic and posthepatic site. The prehepatic causes of PH are portal vein thrombosis, splenic vein thrombosis, arteriovenous fistula, blood overflow in the splanchnic district; the posthepatic causes are the Budd-Chiari syndrome, inferior vena cava obstruction, right-sided heart failure [1]. The liver cirrhosis is a remarkable medical problem in the world. Cirrhosis and hepatic chronic diseases are an important cause of morbidity and mortality worldwide, but with many differences in the geographic distribution. The global mortality rate ranges from 2% to 4% of total deaths in 2017, with decrease from the rate variance 1%–9%, evaluated in 1990 [2]. The more evident clinical evolutions of liver cirrhosis are PH, damage of coagulation, digestive hemorrhage, ascites, hepatic encephalopathy, hepatocarcinoma.

2. PH related gastroduodenal lesions

The PH leads to some pathological conditions in the esophageal and gastroduodenal tract, that can cause digestive hemorrhage. Esophageal varices are the lesion currently developed in the patients with PH by liver cirrhosis or other pre and posthepatic obstacles to splanchnic blood flow. Consequently in these patients all gastrointestinal bleedings are usually ascribed to esophageal varices. Instead others gastroduodenal lesions, potentially hemorrhagic, can be associated with PH. In this group of lesions there are the portal hypertensive gastropathy (PHG), gastric antral vascular ectasia (GAVE), gastric and duodenal ulcer, isolated gastric varices. The aim of this presentation is to evaluate the development, the clinical prominence and therapeutic needs of these lesions, which are associated but also conditioned by PH.

2.1 Portal hypertensive gastropaty

Varices are activated collateral vessels and they develop following the obstruction of portal flow. The role of activation of collateral vessel is to allow the retourn of digestive portal blood flow into the systemic circulation. PHG has similarly its cause in the obstruction in portal flow. All PHG occur in patients with PH, but not all patients with PH can develop PHG. The PHG was previously called as hemorrhagic gastritis within the large group which includes many bleeding gastric pathologies; later it was correctly framed and defined in the context of complications of PH. The clinical observation shows that the patients with severe PH and longer liver disease duration with esophageal varices, expecially if treated with endoscopic procedures, have more frequently PHG. In the gastric mucosa there are congestion and dilated capillaries [3]. The hemodynamic changes of the PH, caused by some mechanical and functional obstacles to portal circulation, as hepatic cirrhosis, pre or posthepatic block, portal hyper-inflow, are the pathophysiological basis of PHG. The congestion of the gastric mucosa is the first phenomenon of the obstruction of the portal flow. The most important question is whether and in which way can occur the change in hematic perfusion of the stomach during PH. The etiology of PHG is not completely known. In the PH there is an important hemodinamic characteristic, that is a hyperdynamic circulation based on the increased hematic flow in the mesenteric, splenic and total gastric sections. The hyperdynamic circulation is one factor which induces the PHG, based on the changes in blood flow of gastric mucosa [4]. The hyperdynamic characteristcs in the PH lead to some important hemodynamic changes in the patients. In the hyperdynamic circulation of PH intrahepatic vascular resistence greaten, whereas mean arterial pressure and systemic vascular resistence reduce and there is wide vasodilatation in the splanchnic sector. Finally the gastric blood flow is globally increased, but the particular gastric mucosal flow should be reduced [5]. The gastric mucosal blood flow, in the patients with PHG, is now discussed. Some studies report decreased gastric mucosal blood flow [6], but these data can be modified, as increase of mucosal blood flow, after correction of PH, for example by TIPS [7]. There are other studies that underline, on the contrary, the increase of gastric mucosal blood flow [8]. Clinical observation in PHG shows major tendency to actions of gastrotoxic substances and decreased wound healing. Consequently the more obvious clinical appearance of PHG is the gastrointestinal bleeding, usualy of mild or moderate entity and diffuse from the gastric wall. Ultimately the hemodynamic changes cause the impairments of gastric mucosal defense competence with major sensitivity to injuries and alteration of growth factors, with minor possibility of mucosal healing [9]. Synthetically the weak gastric mucosa more easily can bleed and reduced mucosal blood perfusion, with altered gastric microcirculation leads to increased sensitivity to hypoxia and noxions agent, with erosion, ulcers and bleeding. PHG is related to severity of liver cirrhosis and in particular is connected with the increase degree of hepatic vein pressure gradient (HVPG). PHG is a dinamic condition because in its evaluation can occur some reversible gastric mucosal changes [10]. PHG incidence raises with increasing of hypertension in the portal area and is associated with esophageal and gastric varices; it's a strong predictor of gastroesophageal varices bleeding [11]. In fact PHG occur frequently in patients with liver cirrhosis and its major incidence is based on the severity of PH. This lesion can modify its degree from midl to severe and can disappear. Bleeding can occur but is not frequent and often of not serious entity. The role of sclerotherapy of esophageal varices on the natural history of PHG is not unanimously defined. Following some experience, the treatment of esophageal varices does not seem to influence the evolution of PHG, but there are others observations opposite to this hipothesis in the literature [12]. PH develops direct action on gastric mucosa. The PHG encompasses a large types of gastric mucosal lesions in the cirrhotic patients. These lesions should be distinguished from others lesions as GAVE, which is an independent pathology. These following modifications shape the PHG. About gastric mucosal hemodinamic changes, it's not clear if gastric mucosal hyperhemia is by active or passive hemodynamic congestion. In the pathogenesis of PHG there are together the action of increase of the portal pressure and of gastric blood flow (hyperdynamic splanchnic circulation) which causes its development. Moreover in PHG there is the damage of gastric mucosal defense factors, with the occurrence of bleeding, that is its unique clinical manifestation [13]. In the pathogenesis of PHG can be identified some steps. The hemodynamic changes in the splanchnic district and in particular in the stomach are caused by increased portal pressure. The most evident modification is the congestion in the gastric wall, with the tissue impairment. Consequently there is the activation of cytokines and growth factors (TNF alfa) and subsequent activation of endothelial constitutive nitric oxide (NO) synthase in the gastric mucosa. The increased presence of NO synthase produces excess of NO which leads to hyperdinamic circulation and overproduction of peroxinitrite, that induces, with endothelin, the major susceptibility of gastric mucosa to injuries [14]. There are controversial data in the literature on the kind of changes of gastric mucosa blood flow: in some studies there is the increase but in others there is decrease of blood flow. In summary remain unclear if hemodynamic changes in PHG are active or passive congestion [15, 16]. Others observations suggest that cirrhotics with PHG have increased gastric perfusion but without congestion. The magnitude of changes in gastric perfusion and the endoscopic severity of PHG had no relationship with the degree of PH [17]. In the patiens with liver cirrhosis can occur both gastric lesions, PHG and GAVE. These pathologies have different pathophysiology and management. They have the same clinical manifestations as gastric bleeding, usually chronic but in some cases the gastric hemorrhage can be acute and with high entity. The endoscopic diagnosis for differentiation can be difficult and the histology can be useful [18]. The endoscopic appearance of the PHG is characteristic: flushed and edematous mucosa that suggest mosaic pattern, dilated mucosal and submucosal vessels without inflammation. Further evolutions of these lesions are friable mucosa which bleeds easily on contact and there are hemorrhagic spots. The site of these pathological mucosal lesions can occur frequently in the proximal stomach, but the same lesions by mesenteric hypertension can be observed in others sections of the gastrointestinal tract [3]. Histological features of PHG are dilated, congested capillaries, edema, extravasated red blood cells (RBCs), smooth muscle hyperplasia [19]. Further special problem is the connection of PHG with infection of Helicobacter pylori (H.pylori). Some data from the literature report that infection prevalence of H.pylori in cirrhotic patients with PHG is lower than general population [20]. The diminution of H.pylori infection in cirrhotic patients should be related to the gastric vascular congestion characteristic of PHG [21]. Mucosal gastric changes in PH are characterized by the alteration of mucus protection, that become slimmer, riduction of gastric acidity based on minor acid secretion, decrease of Prostaglandin with lowered gastric blood flow and impaired gastric barrier. The alteration of gastric mucosal barrier is worsened by severe impairment of gastric wall microcirculation, with the result of vascular congestion, followed by mucosal hypoxia and reduction of oxigen released in gastric mucosa. In summary the debility of gastric mucosal barrier of PHG could make easy mucosal lesions and infectious invasion, e.g. by H.pylori. However the vascular congestion, impaired microcirculation and mucosal hypoxia in PHG allow the increase of intestinal metaplasia of gastric mucosa, which is an opposed element to H.pylory infection [22]. In summary, based on these data of the literature, a current evaluation suggest that the minor H.pylori infection rate in cirrhotic patients with PHG can be connected to intestinal metaplasia of gastric mucosa [23]. Clinical presentation of PHG is the gastrointestinal bleeding. The hemorrhage can present as acute or chronic complication. The frequence of acute bleeding shows a wide range from 2% to more than 40% in various reports [12, 24, 25]. The great variance of frequency can be due to vast time frame of references and to difficulties and imprecisions of endoscopic examination during acute bleeding in congiunction with others potential source hemorrhage as esophageal varices. In summary the endoscopic diagnosis can be sure only if the bleeding point is identified [26]. The acute bleeding in PHG usually, almost 90% of cases, can occur in the patients with advanced cirrhosis, longer duration and major extension and severity of gastropathy. The extent of bleeding in the PHG is usually mild or moderate [27, 28]. Very difficult is the evaluation of the incidence of chronic bleeding from PHG, that frequently can be mild. Some references of the literature report the frequence variation that oscillates between 3%–26% [29]. In fact there are many uncertainties in the definition of chronic bleeding as which level of hemoglobin reduction, but, most important, the coexistent clinical condition of anemia in cirrhotic patients, also without gastrointestinal bleeding. The diagnosis of PHG is only endoscopic. Some endoscopic features have been identified as diagnostic: snake skin, stripped appearance, mild reddening mosaic in the mild appearance of gastropathy; flat red spots, fine red speckling mosaic characterize the endoscopic appearance of moderate disease; finally the more severe condition of gastropathy can be identified in the diffuse hemorrhagic lesions, red spots, point bleeding mosaic. This summary of some classifications proposal of endoscopic features of PHG shows the discordance among various experience reported in the literature, about shared definitions and identifications for each endoscopic lesion of PHG [13, 25, 30]. Most frequently the detection of asymptomatic PHG occur during endoscopic control of esophageal varices in the patients with chronic liver disease. In these patients there is not appearance of gastrointestinal bleeding and you can say that PHG developed spontaneusly. In the evolution of PHG should be evaluated the role of the treatment of esophageal varices by sclerotherapy or ligation. Some data of the literature refer an increased occurrence of PHG following endoscopic therapy of esophageal varices. In this perspective should be proposed prophylactic pharmacotherapy with nonselective betablockers as propranolol. In summary for asymptomatic PHG is usually not required treatment [28, 31]. If the PHG is recognized as the cause of anemia due to chronic bleeding, drug therapy can be started with iron replacement, in some cases blood transfusion and drugs that can lower the pressure in the portal district as betablocker propranolol. In the cases of acute bleeding the first procedures are for the resuscitation of the patient with blood transfusion, vasoconstrictors as somatostatin or analogues and antibiotics. It's suddenly mandatory the endoscopic control of esophageal varices and possible their treatment if bleeding. When there is the endoscopic certainty of PHG as source of acute hemorrhage, should be possible the use of endoscopic therapy also for PHG and the current pharmacotherapy by betablocker propranolol, somatostatin or analogues, vasopressin. In the rare cases of acute hemorrhage not responded to medical therapy can be requested emergency therapy with TIPS [18]. Endoscopic therapy of PHG has been proposed with the use of the laser, but the results are uncertain and consequently it has been little used. All the drugs employed in the management of PHG, connected with hypertensive condition in the portal district are based on the reduction of gastric blood flow and gastric perfusion [3].

2.2 Gastric antral vascular ectasia

Gastric antral vascular ectasia (GAVE) occurs roughly in the 30% of the patients with cirrhosis [32]. Two types of GAVE syndrome, with different natural history and clinical features, can be identified. The non- cirrhotic GAVE syndrome in particurar is associated to autoimmune diseases, more frequently in aged women, with Rainaud's syndrome, sclerodactyly, atrofic gastritis [33]. Beside association with various autoimmune diseases, there are, in non-cirrhotic GAVE syndrome, the pathological association with sclerodermia, chronic renal failure, etc. [34]. The etiology of GAVE syndrome is now yet undefined and the pathogenesis of vascular characteristic alterations as ectasia should by contracted by mechanical actions on the gastric mucosa. This hypothesis is based on some histological characteristics, in particular the fibromuscolar hyperplasia, as results of mechanical actions [35]. The histologic features of GAVE can be summarized with the following data: prevalent presence of the lesions in the antrum, vascular ectasia, submucosal fibrohyalinosis, spindle cells (smooth muscle cell – myofibroblast hyperplasia) proliferation, fibrin thrombi in mucosal vessells [36, 37]. The GAVE syndrome shows the characteristic endoscopic appearance of watermelon stomach, gastric dilation, linear lesions localized in the antrum, vasodilation and tendency to the bleeding. Endoscopic features of GAVE are represented by conglomerates of red spots which are organized in a linear pattern in the gastric antrum, taking shape of watermelon stomach. Following the pathogenetical proposal of Lowes J R, can be evaluated the role of neuroendocrine cells proliferations in GAVE and effect of its vasoactive intestinal peptide on vessels wall with vascular ectasia [38]. The occurrence of GAVE in the patients with liver cirrhosis should be due to the obstacle of the portal flow, consequent PH, spontaneous shunting of mesenteric flow through collateral vessells, as esophageal varices, and impaired hepatic catabolism of some vasoactive substances [35]. The management of GAVE syndrome is not well established in all clinical manifestations. The central aim of the therapeutic procedures is the control of the bleeding, that occurs more frequently in GAVE than in PHG, usually as chronic gastrointestinal hemorrhage, in cirrhotic patients with clinical appearance of chronic anemia. The chronic anemia is a clinical condition that belongs to liver cirrhosis and can be also caused by PHG; for this reason the differential diagnosis of the causes of anemia is necessary to prepare specific therapies [18]. Some procedures have been employed: medical therapies with estrogen and progesterone, tranexamic acid (antifibrinolitic substance), octreotide, propranolol. All these medical treatments showed partial therapeutic effectiveness, therefore, if the ineffective medical therapies, can be accessed to invasive surgical therapies for control of hypertensive condition in mesenteric district, as TIPS or to direct treatment of hemorrhagic source with antrectomy. Unfortunately the surgical procedures in cirrhotic patients can be connected with not negligeable risk of morbidity and mortality [35, 39–41]. In the treatment of GAVE have been employed endoscopic procedures based on thermoablative techniques. In particular argon plasma coagulation and Nd:Yag laser coagulation. For these procedures usually should be repeated some sessions. Cryotherapy has been used with rapid expansion in the stomach of compressed nitroux oxide and following freezing of the mucosa, allowing therapeutic effect on diffuse lesions [42–44]. In the final evaluation we can conclude that endoscopic approach with thermoablative procedures as argon plasma coagulation, Nd:Yag laser coagulation and cryotherapy have advantagious therapeutic effects on decrease of bleeding and needs of blood transusion in complicated hemorrhagic GAVE [18]. In summary PHG and GAVE are potential hemorrhagic mucosal lesions of the stomach that can develop in the patients with PH by liver cirrhosis. Both pathologies can cause more frequently chronic or sometime acute gastrointestinal bleeding. Therefore these conditions have some pathological and clinical differences. The PHG occur only in cirrhotics with PH, the hemorrhagic lesions are located mostly in the gastric fundus and the pharmacological therapies are frequently effective. The GAVE can be also present in the patients without liver cirrhosis and PH (60%–70% of the cases), the gastric site of the lesions is antrum almost always, there is the histological characteristic of fibrin thrombi in the mucosal vessells and signs of mucosal inflammation, finally the therapeutic procedures are endoscopic (argon, laser, cryotherapy).

2.3 Gastric and duodenal ulcer

Another lesions, possible source of upper gastrointestinal bleeding in cirrhotic patients are the peptic ulcers, located in duodenum and stomach. The frequency of bleeding from gastroduodenal ulcers in cirrhotics, rather than from esophageal varices ranges from 5% to 15% [45, 46]. Gastroduodenal peptic ulcer disease maintains a not negligeable prevalence in the general population that reaches 14% [47]. The etiology and natural history of peptic ulcer pathology is connected and conditioned by certain well known factors: mainly environmental, behavioral and infectious, as the infection of H.pylori, curative use of NAIDS, etc. However the role of associated pathologies cannot be left out. In fact liver cirrhosis carries an enlarged risk of occurrence of peptic ulcer disease with the incidence that varies widely from 10% to 49% [48]. The pathophysiological connections among peptic ulcer disease, liver cirrhosis with metabolic changes related and infection of H.pylori are object of numerous studies. Especially the prevalence of H.pylori infection in cirrhotic patients is reported in the various researches with great variability and this does not allow to define if the H.pylori infection has a specific role in the pathogenesis of ulcerative disease in cirrhotics. For example in some studies the high incidence of peptic ulcer in the patients with liver cirrhosis is associated also to great presence of H.pylori infection until 60% of cases [49]. On the other hand there are many studies which refer the prevalence rates of H.pylori infection in cirrhotics not dissimilar compared to the values of non cirrhotic patients [50]. Ultimately the data on the role of H.pylori about the occurrence and development of peptic ulcer during chronic liver disease are debatable and in conclusion uncertain; in any case it's not evident a significant action of H.pylori infection in the pathophysiology of peptic ulcer disease in the cirrhotic patients. Therefore in summary we can believe that there are no significant differences in the prevalence of H.pylori infection between general population and patients with chronic liver disease [50]. Neverthless this observation, it can be accepted that peptic ulcers develop more frequently in the cirrhotic patients. The clinical appearances of peptic ulcers in cirrhotic patients are characterized by negative features of ulcer disease evolution as greater frequence of bleeding and recurrence of the disease and retarded recovery. The reason of greater occurrence of peptic ulcers is based on the modification of gastric-acid secretion, changed gastric mucosal blood flow and, mostly, on damaged mucosal defense mechanisms. In fact there is not evidence of increase of gastric-acid secretion in cirrhotic patients with PH and, on the contrary, the possible variations are almost always as hypocloridric changes likely related to worsening of liver disease [51]. The damaged protective function of gastric mucosal barrier seems to have a greater role in the pathophysiology of peptic ulcers in cirrhotics, based on the occurrence of chronic atrophyc gastritis in liver cirrhosis, the reduced strength of gastric mucosa due to parietal venous congestion and protein and vitamin deficiencies [52]. Others metabolic and functional modifications should integrate the pathogenetic framework of peptic ulcer in cirrhotic patients: raised level of gastrin and histamine, increase of duodenogastric reflux, impaired gastric empting, reduced prostaglandin level in gastric mucosa and decrease of mucosal oxigen saturation [53, 54]. Most recent studies confirm this proposal evaluation referring that the severity degree of liver pathological involvement plays an important role in the development of peptic ulcer disease. Decompensated cirrhosis, the action of PH, more effective if more serious, on gastric mucosal blood flow, on efficiency of mucosal defense barrier and on epithelial resumption, can support ulcer development, the retard of mucosal recovery and possible recurrence of peptic disease [50, 55]. In summary in the pathophysiology of peptic ulcer in cirrhotics, the H.pylori infection and NSAID therapeutic use are risk factors with effects no different than in the general population. However in the patients with cirrhosis and PH, in which peptic ulcer disease occur with notable percentage, the liver pathology operates a significant pathogenetic role [56]. The prevalence of peptic ulcer in cirrhotics is more high compared with general population, both in symptomatic patients with bleeding and in asymptomatic patients [57]. There is a greater prevalence of peptic ulcer disease in cirrhotic patients and these patients have major risk of bleeding from peptic ulcer related to general population; moreover each occurrence of peptic ulcer bleeding is followed by the decompensation of hepatic cirrhosis with increase of severity of clinical conditions [58, 59]. In the patients with liver cirrhosis upper gastrointestinal bleeding is currently reported to esophageal varices, but in the 30% -40% of cases the source of bleeding is not esophageal varices but gastroduodenal ulcers, with subsequent remarkable morbidity and mortality [60]. Upper gastrointestinal bleeding is the common and expected complication of liver cirrhosis with PH. The first therapeutic purpose is to control the hypovolemic alterations of various degrees of severity due to amount of hemorrhage and to steady the hemodynamic conditions. The subsequent step requires by diagnostic approach to differentiate the bleeding from esophageal varices or from others gastroduodenal pathologies connected to hepatic cirrhosis, as peptic ulcers. The hemodynamic instability requires resuscitation, that can be restrictive or aggressive, by infusion of cristalloids (Ringer lactate, normal saline, etc.) or also, in some cases, of colloids (albumin, plasma, dextrane, etc.). If the indication is found can be useful the use of blood transfusion. In the first therapeutic approach the evaluation of bleeding severity encompasses also the assessment of level of the risk of rebleeding in order to graduate the subsequent phases of treatment using Glasgow Blatchford score [61]. The severe gastrointestinal hemorrhage from ulcer lesions in cirrhotic patients adversely affects the prognosis through worsening of already impaired liver functions. In the patients with upper gastrointestinal bleeding from peptic ulcers the therapeutic perspective is based on the pharmacologic treatment that includes the use of proton pump inhibitors, somatostatin and octreotide, and on the endoscopic diagnostic definition and management. The endoscopic therapies, with hemostatic purpose, include various procedures as epinephrine injection, thermocoagulation, sclerosant injection, use of the clips, TC-325 Hemospray. The global management of non variceal upper gastrointestinal bleeding has been recently defined by international guideline [62]. Finally in case of failure of pharmacologic and endoscopic management of peptic ulcers in cirrhotics and serious unmanageable clinical conditions, could be proposed direct surgical gastroduodenal procedures as rescue therapy.

2.4 Isolated gastric varices

Gastric varices are usually connected with esophageal varices, but can be also isolated along the gastric wall. Gastric varices are classified by endoscopy with topographical criterion as gastroesophageal varices type I (lesser gastric curvature), gastroesophageal varices type II (greater gastric curvature); isolated gastric varices type I (gastric fundus), isolated gastric varices type II (any stomach location, except fundus) [63]. The pathogenesis of isolated gastric varices could be ascribed to portal or splenic vein thrombosis. The occurrence of bleeding from isolated gastric varices in the patients with PH shows the percentage incidence from 5% to 10% [64]. The diagnosis of gastric varices is endoscopic. The first general therapeutic approach in the case of bleeding from gastroesophageal or isolated gastric varices is included within the current management of gastrointestinal hemorrhage in the PH, by pharmacological and endoscopic procedures, or portosystemic derivation procedures as TIPS. The specific treatment of isolated gastric varices bleedind is endoscopic usually by injection with cyanoacrylate [65].

3. Conclusions

In the clinical scenario of gastroduodenal lesions associated with PH and liver cirrhosis, both are important actors, but the PH and hepatic chronic disease remain the protagonist of the clinical state. In fact the degree of functional hepatic impairment and of hypertensive status in the splanchnic district affect much the patients general conditions. Moreover the upper gastrointestinal bleeding is the more frequent complication of this complex pathological condition. Esophageal varices currently develop in the cirrhotics with PH and this is the characteristic source of gastrointestinal bleeding. However upper digestive hemorrhage in cirrhotic patients alwais requires the diagnostic definition of bleeding source, which may also be due to pathologies related to PH. In fact, albeit less frequently, others gastroduodenal lesions, with pathogenetic association to liver cirrhosis and PH, may present intestinal hemorrhage. The PHG is in several cases neglected complication of liver cirrhosis and PH. PHG is connected with the degree of PH and can have a role as prognostic index of liver cirrhosis. The management of PHG is based on pharmacological, endoscopic or, in some few cases, on emergency therapy with TIPS. GAVE can affect one third of cirrhotics. PHG and GAVE may both occur in patients with liver cirrhosis. However these pathologies have different pathophysiology and management. The central diagnostic aim is to distinguish GAVE from PHG because the therapeutic procedures that allow decrease of portal pressure, effective for PHG, are not efficacious therapy for GAVE, usually treated by endoscopic approach. Gastric and duodenal ulcer are more frequent in cirrhotics and may worsen prognosis. Early diagnosis and treatment of peptic ulcer in cirrhotic patients are significant to avoid complications. Gastric varices, usually connected with esophageal varices, can be, in some cases, isolated; their therapeutic approach in case of bleeding is enclosed within the effective management of gastrointestinal hemorrhage in the PH. In conclusion the complete diagnosis that identifies with certainty, the bleeding source is decisive for the therapeutic choices.

Author details

Vincenzo Neri*, Nicola Tartaglia, Alberto Fersini, Pasquale Cianci, Mario Pacilli, Giovanna Pavone and Antonio Ambrosi
General Surgery, Department of Medical and Surgical Sciences, University of Foggia, Italy

*Address all correspondence to: vincenzo.neri@unifg.it

References

[1] Bloom S, Kemp W, Lubel J. Portal hypertension: pathophysiology, diagnosis and management. Internal Medicine Journal 2015;45:16-26.

[2] GBD 2017 Cirrhosis Collaborators. The global, regional and national burden of cirrhosis by cause in 195 countries and territories, 1990-2017: a systematic analysis for the Global Burden of Disease Study 2017. Lancet Gastroenterol Hepatol 2020;5:245-266.

[3] Wong F. Portal hypertensive gastropathy. Gastroenter Hepatol 2007;3:428-430.

[4] Gjeorgjievski M, Cappell MS. Portal hypertensive gastropathy: a systematic review of the pathophysiology, clinical presentation, natural history and therapy. World J Hepatol 2016;8:231-262.

[5] Blendis L, Wong F. The hyperdynamic circulation in cirrhosis: an overview. Pharmacol Ther. 2001;89:221-231.

[6] Vyas K, Gala B, Sawant P. et al. Assessment of portal hemodynamics by ultrasound color doppler and laser doppler velocimetry in liver cirrhosis. Indian J Gastroenterol 2002;21:176-178.

[7] Mezawa S, Homma H, Ohta H. et al. Effect of transjugular intrahepatic portosystemic shunt formation on portal hypertensive gastropathy and gastric circulation. Am J Gastroenterol 2001;96:1155-1159.

[8] Shigenuri H, Iwao T, Ikegami M. et al. Effect of propanolol on gastric mucosal perfusion and serom gastric level in cirrhotic patients with portal hypertensive gastropathy. Dig Dis Sci 1994;39:2433-2438.

[9] Perini RF, Camara PRF, Ferraz JGP. Pathogenesis of portal hypertensive gastropathy: traslatic basic research into clinical practice. Nat Clin Pract Gastroenterol Hepatol 2009;6:150-158.

[10] Bang SC, Kim HS, Suk KT. Et al. Portal hypertensive gastropathy as a prognostic index in patients with liver cirrhosis. BMC Gastroenterology 2016;16:93.

[11] Burak KW, Beck PL. Portal hypertensive gastropathy and GAVE syndrome. GUT 2001;49:866-872.

[12] Parmignani M, Carpinelli L, Preatoni P. et al. Natural history of portal hypertensive gastropathy in patients with liver cirrhosis. Gastroenterology 2000;119:181-187.

[13] Eleftheriadis E. Portal hypertensive gastropathy. A clinically significant puzzle. Am Gastroenterol 2001;14:196-204.

[14] Ohta M, Ymaguchi S, Gotoh N. et al. Pathogenesis of portal hypertensive gastropathy. A clinical and experimental review. Surgery 2002;131:S165-S170.

[15] Ohta M, Hashizume M, Higashi H. et al. Portal and gastric hemodynamics in cirrhotic patients with portal hypertensive gastropathy. Hepatology 1994;20:1432-1436.

[16] Iwao T, Toyonaga A, Ikegami M. et al. Reduced gastric mucosal blood flow in patients with portal hypertensive gastropathy. Hepatology 1993;18:36-40.

[17] Panes J, Bordas JM, Piquè JM, et al. Increased gastric mucosal perfusion in cirrhotic patients with portal hypertensive gastropathy. Gastroenterology 1992;103:1875-1882.

[18] Ripoll C, Garcia-Tsao G. The management of portal hypertensive gastropathy and gastric antral vascular

ectasia. Digestive and liver Disease 2011;43:345-351.

[19] Chandamwale SS, Gupta N, Sheth J et al. Histopathological study of portal hypertensive gastropathy using gastric biopsies. Med J DY Patil Vidyapeeth 2017;10:562-567.

[20] Grassi M, Schiffino L, Messini F, et al. Endoscopic and histologic findings of gastric mucosa and Helicobacter pylori prevalence in patients suffering from chronic liver disease. Clin Ter 1996;147:117-122.

[21] Parikh SS, Desai SB, Trivedi MH, et al. Congestive gastropathy: factors influencing development endoscopic features, Helicobacter pylori infection and microvessel change. Am J Gastroenterol 1994;89:1036-1042.

[22] Ibrisim D, Cevikbas U, Akyuz F, et al. Intestinal metaplasia in portal hypertensive gastropathy: a frequent pathology. Eur J Gastroenterol Hepatol 2008;20:874-880.

[23] Hu JK, Li XM, Gu BH, et al. Helicobacter pylori and portal hypertensive gastropathy. Hepatobiliary Pancreatic Diseases International 2018;17:578-580.

[24] Stewart CA, Sanyal AJ. Grading portal gastropathy: validation of a gastropathy scoring system. Am J Gastroenterol 2003;98:1758-1765.

[25] McCormack TT, Sims J, Eyre-Brook I, et al. Gastric lesions in portal hypertension: inflammatory gastritis or congestive gastropathy? GUT 1985;26:1226-1232.

[26] Thuluvath PJ, Yoo HY. Portal hypertensive gastropathy. Am J Gastroenterol 2002;97:2973-2978.

[27] Cubillas R, Rockey DC. Portal hypertensive gastropathy: a review. Liver Int 2010;30:1094-1102.

[28] Sarin SK, Shahi HM, Jain M, et al. The natural history of portal hypertensive gastropathy: influence of variceal eradication Am J Gastroenterol 2000;95:2888-2893.

[29] Merli M, Nicolini G, Angeloni S, et al. The natural history of portal hypertensive gastropaty in patients with liver cirrhosis and mild portal hypertension. Am J Gastroenterol 2004;99:1959-1965.

[30] Tatoue K, Hashizume M, Wada H, et al. Effects of endoscopic injection sclerotherapy on portal hypertensive gastropathy: a prospective study. Gastrointest Endosc 1992;38:582-585.

[31] El-Khayat HR, El-Khattib A, Nasseir M, et al. Portal hypertensive gastropathy before and after variceal obliteration: an endoscopic, histopathologic and immunohistochemical study. J Gastrointest Liver Dis. 2010;19:175-179.

[32] Payen JL, Cales P. Gastric modifications in cirrhosis. Gastroenterol Clin Biol. 1991;15:285-295.

[33] Gostout CJ, Viggiano TR, Ahlquist DA, et al. The clinical and endoscopic spectrum of the watermelon stomach. J Clin Gastroenterol 1992;15:256-263.

[34] Murphy FT, Enzenaner RJ, Cheney CP. Watermelon stomach. Arthritis Rheum 1999;42:573.

[35] Spahr L, Villeneuve JP, Dufresne MP, et al. Gastric antral vascular ectasia in cirrhotic patients: absence of relation with portal hypertension. GUT 1999;44:739-742.

[36] Payen JL, Cales P, Voigt JJ, et al. Severe portal hypertensive gastropathy and antral vascular ectasia are distinct entities in patients with cirrhosis. Gastroenterology 1995;108:138-144.

[37] Gilliam JH, Geisinger RR, Wu WC, et al. Endoscopic biopsy is diagnostic in gastric antral vascular ectasia. The watermelon stomach. Dig Dis Sci 1989;34:885-888.

[38] Lowes JR, Rode J. Neuroendocrine cell proliferations in gastric antral vascular ectasia. Gastroenterology 1989;97:207-212.

[39] Gostout JC, Ahlquist DA, Radford CM, et al. Endoscopic laser therapy for watermelon stomach. Gastroenterology 1989;96:1462-1465.

[40] Manning JR. Estrogen-Progesterone treatment of diffuse antral vascular ectasia. Am J Gastroenterol 1995;90:154-156.

[41] Park RH, Danesh BJ, Upadhyay R, et al. Gastric antral vascular ectasia (watermelon stomach): therapeutic options. Postgrad Med J 1990;66:720-723.

[42] Izquierdo S, Rey E, Gutierrez Del Olmo A, et al. Polyp as a complication of argon plasma coagulation in watermelon stomach. Endoscopy 2005;37:921.

[43] Dulai GS, Jensen DM, Kovacs TO, et al. Endoscopic treatment outcomes in watermelon stomach patients with or without portal hypertension. Endoscopy 2004;36:68-72.

[44] Cho S, Zanati S, Yong E, et al. Endoscopic cryotherapy for the management of gastric antral vascular ectasia. Gastrointest Endosc 2008;68:895-902.

[45] Shahnin WA, Abdel-Baset EZ, Nasser AK, et al. Low incidence of Helicobacter pylori in patients with duodenal ulcer and chronic liver disease. Scand J Gastroenterol 2001;36:479-484.

[46] Nasir N. Esophageal varices vs peptic ulcer a study of 100 patients presenting in Mayo Hospital with upper gastrointestinal bleeding. Pakistan J Gastroenterol 1998;2:58-63.

[47] Del Valle J, Chey WD, Scheiman JM. Acid peptic disorders. In Yamada T, Alpers DH eds. Textbook of Gastroenterology 4th ed. Philadelphia, Lippincot Williams and Wilkins; 2003:1322-1376.

[48] Vergara M, Calvet X, Roque M. Helicobacter pylori is a risk factor for peptic ulcer disease in cirrhotic patients: a meta-analysis. Eur J Gastroenterol Hepatol 2002;14:717-722.

[49] Dore PM, Mura D, Deledda S, et al. Active peptic ulcer disease in patients with hepatitis C virus-related cirrhosis: the role of Helicobacter pylori infection and portal hypertensive gastropathy. Can J Gastroenterol 2004;18:521-524.

[50] Aurux J, Lamarque D, Roudot-Thoravel F, et al. Gastroduodenal ulcer and erosions are related to portal hypertensive gastropathy and recent alcohol intake in cirrhotic patients. Dig Dis Sci 2003;48:1118-1123.

[51] Christensen E, Fanesholdt L, Schlichting P, et al. Aspects of the natural history of gastrointestinal bleeding in cirrhosis and the effect of prednisone. Gastroenterology 1981; 81:944-952.

[52] Ferrarese S, Neri V, Pranzo L. Ipertensione portale e lesioni gastroduodenali associate. In Fisiopatologia Chirurgica. Ferrarese S Ed. Il Pensiero Scientifico Editore. Roma. 1985:273-276.

[53] Tanaka M, Inatsuchi S, Terrasaki T, et al. Duodenal mucosal hemodynamics in patients with liver cirrhosis. Acta Med Okayama 1990;44:273-277.

[54] Al Amri SM. Frequency of peptic ulcers in patients with portal

hypertension. Ann Saudi Med 1995;15:451-454.

[55] Kitano S, Dolgor B. Does portal hypertension contribute to the pathogenesis of gastric ulcer associated with liver cirrhosis? J Gastroenterol 2000;35:79-86.

[56] Saad RJ, Chey WD. Peptic ulcer disease in patients with chronic liver disease: looking beyond bugs and drugs. Gastrointest Endosc 2005;62:357-359.

[57] Voulgaris T, Karagiannakis D, Siakavellas S et al. High prevalence of asymptomatic peptic ulcers diagnosed during screening endoscopy in patient with cirrhosis. Ann Gastroenterol 2019;32:1-6.

[58] Kirchner GI, Beil W, Blek JS et al. Prevalence of Helicobacter pylori and occurrence of gastroduodenal lesions in patients liver cirrhosis. Int J Clin Exp Med 2011;4:26-31.

[59] Luo JC, Leu HB, Hou MC, et al. Cirrhotic patients at increased risk of peptic ulcer bleeding: a nationwide population-based cohort study. Aliment Pharmacol Ther 2012;36:542-550.

[60] Gonzales J, Garcia-Compean D, Vazquez-Elizondo G, et al. Nonvariceal upper gastrointestinal bleeding in patients with liver cirrhosis. Clinical features, outcomes and predictors of in-hospital mortality: A prospective study. Ann Hepatol 2011;10:287-295.

[61] Laursen SB, Dalton HR, Murray IA, et al. Upper Gastrointestinal Hemorrhage International Consortium. Performance of new thresholds of the Glasgow Blatchford score in managing patients with upper gastrointestinal bleeding. Clin Gastroenterol Hepatol 2015;13:115-121.

[62] Barkun AN, Almadi M, Kuipers EJ, et al. Management of non variceal upper gastrointestinal bleeding: guideline raccomandations from the International Consensus Group. Ann Int Med 2019:1-23. Doi.org/10.7326/M19-1795.

[63] Sarin SK, Lahoti D, Soxena SP, et al. Prevalence classification and natural history of gastric varices: a long-term follow-up study in 568 portal hypertension patients. Hepatology 1992;16:1343-1349.

[64] Bosch J, Abraldes JG, Groszmznn. Current management of portal hypertension. J Hepatol Suppl 2003;38:S54-S68.

[65] Sarin SK, Jain AK, Jain M, et al. A randomized controlled trial of cyanoacrylate versus alcohol injection in patient with isolated fundic varices. Am J Gastroenterol 2002;97:1010-1015.

Chapter 9

Anaesthetic Considerations in Gastrointestinal Endoscopies

Moad Ali M. Ehfeda, Adel Ganaw,
Sohel Mohamed Gamal Ahmed, Arshad Chanda, Zia Mahood,
Salem Jabira, Hossam Algallie, Ahmad H.M. Almaqadma,
Mahmud M.A. Ben Masoud, Ali O. Mohamed Bel Khair
and Qazi Zeeshan

Abstract

Gastrointestinal endoscopy has become fundamental procedure for diagnosis and treatment of gastrointestinal tract diseases. Generally, the gastrointestinal endoscopy is minimally invasive procedure. However, it can cause considerable amount of discomfort and pain which make the procedure unsafe, complicated and refusal of follow up procedures if done without safe sedation. The sedation is required to alleviate anxiety, provide analgesia, amnesia and to improve endoscopic performance specifically in therapeutic procedures. The safe administration of sedative and analgesic medications, irrespective of the regimen used, requires knowledge of the individual needs of patients. The combination of benzodiazepines and opioids is now the most widely used sedation regimen for sedation in gastrointestinal endoscopic procedures. Generally, sedation for gastrointestinal endoscopy is considered safe, however, it has the potential for serious complications. Therefore, endoscopist should assess the patients properly before the endoscopy as well as should be aware of all possible complications and the risk factors. Furthermore, skilled staff and emergency equipment should be available in endoscopy suit. This chapter discuss in details all the aspects of safe procedural sedation during GI endoscopies.

Keywords: sedation, analgesia, gastrointestinal endoscopy, monitoring

1. Introduction

With the advancement in the field of medicine there is a consistent increase in number of diagnostic and therapeutic procedures which are done as day care basis. These procedures can cause considerable amount of discomfort and pain which make the procedure unsafe, complicated and refusal of follow up procedures if done without safe sedation. The GI endoscopies are a kind of procedures that need sedation to facilitate the procedures, alleviate discomfort, pain and eventually making them safe and successful.

Sedation is drug induced depression of the conscious level; it is also call as procedural sedation. Sedation is a continuum ranging from minimal sedation i.e., anxiolysis, moderate sedation (also known as Conscious sedation), Deep sedation and finally general anesthesia. Sedation for GI endoscopy needs proper planning like preprocedural preparation, risk assessment, focus physical examination and optimization of comorbid condition if any. Other considerations in the sedation managements like the selection of a suitable sedation, analgesia regimen depends on the type and duration of procedure, patient and endoscopist satisfaction and last not the least on the competency of the provider. Monitoring during procedure is one of the crucial points in the safe sedation practice. The post procedure care is an essential part of patient safety which need monitoring of the patient in the recovery area where the adverse events secondary to the procedure or the sedation can be discovered and addressed promptly.

2. Definition

Sedation is the depression in the perception of patient's surroundings, leading to the decrease of his or her reactivity to external stimuli [1]. Sedation seldomly occurs without different degrees of related effects of sedative agents which may be dose-dependent, such as:

- Anxiolysis: Relieve of apprehension or agitation with limited sensory alteration.
- Amnesia: loss of consciousness for a period of time.
- Analgesia: pain relief without a change in level of consciousness.
- Anesthesia: loss of consciousness.
- Sedation has been a common addition to modern medical care as a means of promoting complicated or painful procedures in a safe, cost-effective and time-saving alternative to general anesthesia.

The endoscopist must completely comprehend the sedation being used. Patient factors, the setup of the GI endoscopy service and the variables of the procedure itself are to be carefully considered. Age, weight, medical history, concurrent drugs, airway anatomy, preprocedural anxiety and pain tolerance are patient variables. The amount of expected pain, the length of the test, and how invasive the procedure would be are examples of procedural variables.

The area of the endoscopy suite, the ease of staff moving around, the presence of emergency airway management equipment, the different level of skills of personnel present and whether the procedure is carried out in a hospital setting or in a stand-alone clinic are all important part of the setup.

3. Sedation levels

In recent years, four levels of sedation have been established that extend along a spectrum without clear limits: minimal sedation or anxiolysis, moderate sedation, deep sedation, and general anesthesia [1]. These sedation levels have been characterized by the reaction of a patient to verbal, light contact, or painful stimuli, although they are often associated with physiological changes in vital patient signs.

"Minimal sedation" is also known as anxiolysis and is defined as the lowest drug-induced stage of cognition-impairment. Individuals who are minimally sedated usually respond to simple orders and their breathing/cardiovascular system is unaffected. Oral benzodiazepines are commonly used to achieve minimal sedatives.

"Moderate Sedation" has traditionally been referred to as "Conscious Sedation". This entitles a deeper depression consciousness level. Individuals who are moderately sedated can still respond to verbal orders, often requiring physical stimulation, and their breathing/cardiovascular function is unaffected. Intravenous benzodiazepines and opioids are examples of drugs used to achieve moderate sedation.

'Deep sedation' leads to major depression of the central nervous system, where patients are no longer conscious and are more difficult to arouse. They will usually respond to painful stimuli but not to verbal or simple tactile stimuli. The respiratory system is stressed and some ventilatory assistance may be required.

Intravenous benzodiazepines, intravenous anesthetics such as propofol, ketamine, etomidate, and dexmedetomidine are examples of medicines used for deep sedation.

'General anesthesia' is the deepest type of sedation in which there is a total lack of consciousness and no response to stimuli. Cardiovascular and respiratory functions are often compromised, therefore, monitoring and assistance, such as ventilatory support, may be needed.

A fifth level/form of sedation, also known as 'Dissociative sedation is a variant of moderate sedation characteristically produced by a medication class known as phencyclidine, such as ketamine, which induces a disconnection between the thalamo-neocortical system and the limbic structures, preventing sensory stimuli from being received by higher centers [2, 3].

4. Sedation indications

In most countries, procedural sedation and analgesia (PSA) is common practice in order to promote the success and ease of different diagnostic and therapeutic procedures which do not need muscle paralysis.

Alongside gastroenterology, many other medical disciplines, such as cardiology, gynecology, dentistry, radiology, dermatology, plastic surgery, and emergency medicine, are currently using PSA, and the list is ever expanding. The primary clinician and the patient make a mutual decision to carry out the procedure under PSA.

5. Principles of safe procedural sedation and analgesia

Most procedural sedation occur outside and far from operating theaters; others might occur in standalone clinics outside hospitals. This constitutes a risk, as should an airway emergency happen, anesthetists and other experts in airway management are usually not available to hand. Other emergencies such as cardiac arrests have been extensively reported in the medical literature. Based on above, it is paramount that patients selected for these procedures are carefully evaluated and stratified. A lot of emphasis should be put on airway assessment of these patients and if there is any doubt, they must be referred to a qualified anesthetist for further evaluation and classification.

5.1 Pre-procedure patient assessment

The first stage of secure sedation practice is the proper selection of patients for sedation. To assess his or her suitability for sedation outside the operating room, each patient must be explicitly evaluated.

Patient selection requires collecting patient information as well as supplying the patient with information. The retrieval and review of previous documents, i.e. medical, sedation, anesthesia and surgical history, should be included in pre-assessment wherever possible. Pre-procedural assessment should include history, examinations and laboratory investigations.

5.1.1 Preoperative history

The Preoperative history should include the patient's medical problems and the intended investigative or therapeutic procedure. History of chronic disease, severity and chronic medications should be investigated. Because of the possibility of drug interactions with anesthesia full medication history include using alcohol, tobacco, marijuana, cocaine, herbal medications, and psychotropic drugs sedatives, anxiolytics, antidepressants, antipsychotics, antiepileptics, and drugs used in the treatment of mania) should obtained from every patient. Previous allergic history should be elicited.

Furthermore, detailed history of previous sedation and anesthesia may disclose the previous perioperative challenges such as difficulty in airway management, aspiration, post-operative intensive care admission which may suggest unsuitability of such patients for out of hospital procedures. In addition, general review of organ system may be useful to identify undiagnosed problems.

5.1.2 Physical examination

Although, proper history direct the treating physician to perform focus examination, the physical examination is extremely important to detect abnormalities not obvious in the history. Both history and physical examination complement one another.

General examination should include minimally measurements of vital signs (Blood pressure, heart rate, respiratory rate and temperature), airway evaluation, cardiovascular and respiratory system examination.

5.1.2.1 Airway examination

Sedation practitioner should inspect patient's dentition for denture, bridges or loose teeth. Difficulty in mask ventilation and airway should be anticipated in edentulous as well as those with significant facial abnormalities such as micrognathia, prominent upper incisors, macroglossia, limited mouth opening, short neck, and limited neck mobilities. There are variety of airway reliable assessment scales such as upper lip bite test (ULBT) (**Table 1**) and Mallampati scale (**Table 2**) have been proposed to assist anesthesiologist and sedation practitioner to assist the airway. **Figures 1** and **2** [5].

Classes	Discerption
Class I	lower incisors can bite the upper lip above the vermilion line.
Class II	lower incisors can bite the upper lip below the vermilion line.
Class III	lower incisors cannot bite the upper lip.

Table 1.
Upper lip bite test (ULBT).

Classes	Visible structures	Predicted intubation
Class 1	soft palate, fauces, uvula and pillars	Easy
Class 2	soft palate, fauces and base of uvula	Easy
Class 3	soft palate	Difficult
Class4	hard palate	Difficult

Table 2.
Mallampati score.

5.1.2.1.1 Upper lip bite test (ULBT)

ULBT is one of the several bedside tests used for prediction of difficult intubation, it is performed by asking the patient to bite the upper lip (**Table 1**, **Figure 1**) [6].

5.1.2.1.2 Mallampati classifications

The Mallampati Classification is extremely useful in detection of potential obstructive sleep apnea as well as predictions of difficult endotracheal intubation,

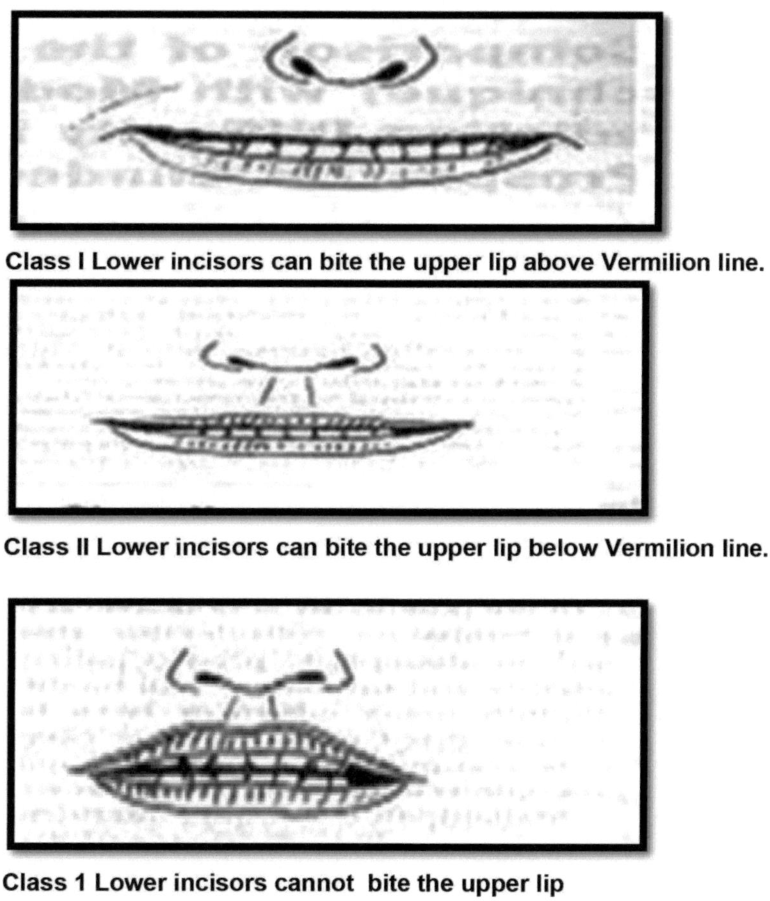

Figure 1.
ULBT.

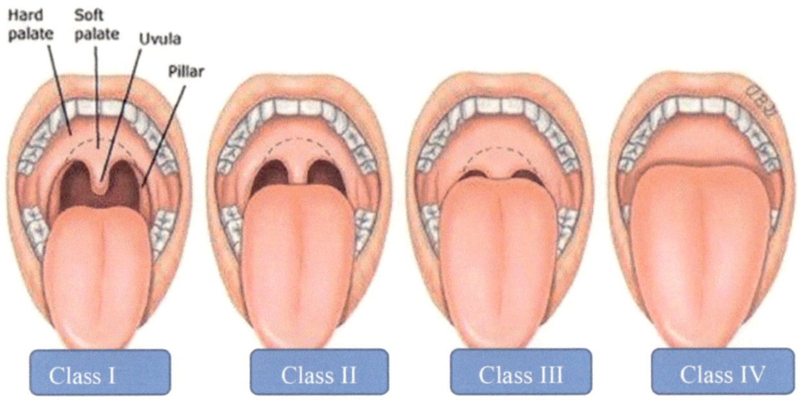

Figure 2.
Mallampati score [4].

The mallampati score is based on the visibility of the pharyngeal structures with maximal mouth opening and tongue protrusion in the setting position (**Table 2**, **Figure 2**).

5.1.3 Laboratory investigations

If the history and clinical examination fail to detect any abnormalities, routine investigations for healthy asymptomatic patients is not recommended as it increases the cost, delay the procedure and rarely changes the perioperative management. Therefore, investigations should be obtained only for specific clinical indication and for patients in whom the abnormality may be expected.

Pregnancy test may be considered for fertile women to avoid potential teratogenic effect for sedative agents on fetus in case of undiagnosed pregnancy.

5.1.4 ASA physical status classification

A re-evaluation of health status shortly before sedation and surgery is advised if the patient has been seen at an earlier appointment. The evaluation should be performed in accordance with the Physical Status Classification Scheme of the American Society of Anesthesiologists (ASA) (**Table 3**) [7]. Although the ASA classification is used by anesthesia and sedation suppliers to denote the overall preoperative status of a patient for anesthesia and sedation, a risk prediction cluster can be confused. It is necessary to note that this is not a classification of risk, but rather a clinical status assessment. For sedation outside the operating room, only patients in ASA Class I and II should be considered. ASA Class III, IV or V patients need higher levels of supervision and treatment. These patients are recommended to be carried out in-hospital.

5.2 Categories of patients that need special treatment include

5.2.1 Obese patient

Sedating the obese patients, especially out of hospital setting where the resources are limited is challenging to all sedative practitioners. Clinical assessment of functional capacity and myocardial functions of obese patient is not reliable due to sedentary life style and restricted physical activities. In addition, most of the obese patients suffer from chronic diseases such as diabetes mellites, hypertension, obstructive sleep apnea, and pulmonary hypertension which make

DOI: http://dx.doi.org/10.5772/intechopen.96687

ASA PS Classification	Definition	Adult Examples, Including, but not Limited to:	Pediatric Examples, Including but not Limited to:	Obstetric Examples, Including but not Limited to:
ASA I	A normal healthy patient	Healthy, non- smoking, no or minimal alcohol use	Healthy (no acute or chronic disease), normal BMI percentile for Age	
	A patient	Mild diseases only	Asymptomatic	Normal pregnancy*, well
	with mild	Without	Congenital	controlled gestational HTN,
	Systemic	substantive	cardiac disease,	controlled preeclampsia
	Disease	functional	well controlled	without severe features,
		limitations. Current	dysrhythmias,	diet-controlled gestational
		smoker, social	asthma without	DM.
		alcohol drinker,	exacerbation,	
ASA II		pregnancy, obesity (30 < BMI < 40),	well controlled epilepsy, non-	
		well-controlled	Insulin	
		DM/HTN, mild	Dependent	
		lung disease	Diabetes	
			mellitus,	
			abnormal BMI	
			percentile for	
			age,mild/moderate OSA, oncologic state in remission, autism with mild limitations	

ASA PS Classification	Definition	Adult Examples, Including, but not Limited to:	Pediatric Examples, Including but not Limited to:	Obstetric Examples, Including but not Limited to:
ASA III	A patient with severe systemic disease	Substantive Functional limitations; One or more moderate to severe diseases. Poorly controlled DM or HTN, COPD, morbid obesity (BMI ≥40), active hepatitis, Alcohol dependence or abuse, implanted pacemaker, Moderate reduction of ejection fraction, ESRD undergoing regularly scheduled dialysis, history (>3 months) of MI, CVA, TIA, or CAD/stents.	Uncorrected Stable Congenital Cardiac abnormality, asthma with exacerbation, poorly controlled epilepsy, insulin Dependent Diabetes mellitus, morbid obesity, malnutrition, severe OSA, oncologic state, renal failure, Muscular dystrophy, cystic fibrosis, history of organ transplantation, brain/spinal cord malformation, Symptomatic hydrocephalus, premature infant PCA <60 weeks, autism with severe limitations, Metabolic disease, difficult airway, long term parenteral nutrition. Full term infants <6 weeks of age.	Preeclampsia with severe features, gestational DM with complications or high insulin requirements, a thrombophilic disease requiring anticoagulation.
ASA IV	A patient with severe systemic disease that is a constant threat to life	Recent (<3 months) MI, CVA, TIA or CAD/stents, ongoing cardiac ischemia or severe valve dysfunction, severe reduction of ejection fraction, shock, sepsis, DIC, ARD or ESRD not undergoing regularly scheduled dialysis	Symptomatic Congenital cardiac abnormality, congestive heart failure, active sequelae of prematurity, acute hypoxic-ischemic encephalopathy, shock, sepsis, disseminated intravascular coagulation, automatic implantable cardioverter- defibrillator, ventilator dependence, endocrinopathy, severe trauma, severe respiratory distress, advanced oncologic state.	Preeclampsia with severe features complicated by HELLP or other adverse event, peripartum cardiomyopathy with EF <40, uncorrected/decompensated heart disease, acquired or congenital.
ASA V	A moribund patient who is not expected to survive without the operation	Ruptured abdominal/thoracic aneurysm, massive trauma, intracranial bleed with mass effect, ischemic bowel in the face of significant cardiac pathology or multiple organ/system dysfunction	Massive trauma, intracranial hemorrhage with mass effect, patient requiring ECMO, respiratory failure or arrest, malignant hypertension, decompensated congestive heart failure, hepatic encephalopathy, ischemic bowel or multiple organ/system dysfunction.	Uterine rupture.
ASA VI	A declared brain-dead patient whose organs are being removed from donor purposes			

Table 3.
ASA physical status classification.

these group of patients are not candidate for day case surgery or out of hospital setting. Sedative, anesthetics and opioid promote pharyngeal collapse, airway obstruction and alter normal respiratory response to obstruction and apnea in patients who suffer from obstructive sleep apnea which might increase the jeopardy of mortality and morbidity. Moreover, obese patients have significant reduction in functional residual capacity and rapidly desaturated [8]. Establishment of intravenous access, airway management, positioning and monitoring of obese patients are extremely difficult and require well trained sedative practitioners as well as immediate help.

5.2.2 Elderly patients

The patient's upper age limit for outside-hospital procedures should be individually defined. The decision is based on considerations such as the invasiveness and length of the procedure, comorbidity, chronic medications and whether there is aftercare at home. Patients older than 65 years of age should be carefully selected for potential reduced organ function and increased occurrence of co-existing diseases. These patients often have limited reserves and can become degraded more rapidly and have more cardiac events. There is a strong correlation between advanced age and median successful dose reduction for all central nervous system medications regardless rout of administration.

5.2.3 Pregnancy

Gastrointestinal endoscopy in pregnant women should only be carried out if it's strongly indicated and deferred to the second trimester wherever possible.

The pregnant woman should be properly aware of the essence of the procedure, the possible advantages and complications, including the risks resulting from sedative medications, on herself and the fetus, and should take a fully informed decision. Whenever possible, procedures should be carried out without any sedation, thus preventing ventilatory dysfunction as well as subsequent hypoxemia and potential teratogenicity. In situations where sedation is inevitable, a minimum clinically appropriate dosage must be maintained for sedative agents. Further advices involve maternal and fetal monitoring during endoscopy, and putting the patient in a lateral decubitus position, to avoid the vena caval and aortic compression through the gravid uterus, and applying the bipolar current to electrocoagulation.

Teratogenic effects of propofol and fentanyl in humans have never been proved conclusively and these agents have strong safety records in appropriate pregnant doses. While a correlation between benzodiazepine use and oral cleft abnormalities has been identified, this finding has not been verified by later case–control studies. Since the duration of organogenesis is during the first trimester of pregnancy, it is widely advised that all but truly emergency endoscopic procedures requiring sedation be delayed until later in pregnancy in order to prevent possible teratogenicity. A meta-analysis of anesthetic exposure studies during pregnancy concluded that the only potential issue concerning general-anesthetic exposure is a small increase in the incidence of miscarriage. Although most current anesthetic and analgesic agents cross the placental barrier to varying degrees, their possible adverse fetal effects tend to be limited a and if administered judiciously, are well tolerated by the fetus. It should be stressed, however, that all the published recommendations are backed by minimal evidence, especially in the case of colonoscopy, and that adherence to those recommendations could not guarantee an uneventful course of pregnancy and the development of the fetus [9, 10].

5.2.4 Children

Pediatric patients are less supportive than adult patients, and their parents also feel more anxiety about the procedure. The effect of sedation varies according to the age of pediatric patients [11]. Children below the age of 6 months may have little anxiety and may be easily affected by sedation. Patients who are six months of age or older, however, have already developed unusual anxiety and will require that their parents stay with them during induction. For children of school age, sedating them is surprisingly challenging as they have developed concrete thinking. As a result, to minimize their level of discomfort, it is advised to carefully address what to expect during the operation.

5.3 Fasting guidelines

Preoperative fasting prior to a procedure carried under sedation is contentious. Some authorities regard it as unnecessary, especially in dentistry and emergency medicine; the idea being Airway protective reflexes are intact during mild and moderate sedation but may be lost during deep sedation. However, if deep sedation is planned, via dissociative or non-dissociative techniques, the following fasting duration recommendations should be followed: [12].

- 2 hours from the last ingestion of breast milk
- 4 hours from the ingestion of Formula for infants
- 6 hours from the consumption of nonhuman milk
- 2 hours from last intake of Clear liquids (defined as fluid without particles e.g. apple juice)
- 6 hours from any solid food intake:

In situations where mild to moderate sedation fails to facilitate the procedure, and the patient is not adequately fasting as above, the procedure should be halted. In an emergency, a general anesthetic can be considered with a rapid sequence induction technique.

6. Procedure monitoring

The Academy of Medical Royal Colleges in Safe Sedation Practice for Healthcare Procedures describes the principles of monitoring during and after the procedure. All sedation team members shall have a comprehensive knowledge of monitoring equipment and an interpretation of the information provided by monitoring devices.

The sedation technique employed is to decide what degree of monitoring is appropriate. This means either basic/standard sedation or advanced sedation.

During basic/standard techniques in which only one individual pharmacological agent is used, respiratory and cardiovascular systems typically are not affected. The intermittent examination of vital signs, e.g. sedation level, anxiety, skin color and breathing habits, is sufficient. A pulse oximetric and non-invasive blood pressure monitor are mandatory for extended procedures [13, 14].

When advanced sedation methods are deployed, the following must be controlled and documented:

1. **Levels and actions of distress** such as agitation and restlessness: This can suggest potential adverse events, such as hypoxemia, hypoglycemia, under-sedation or even over-sedation.

2. **In controlling the level of sedation;** frequent contact with the patient will help. A significant part of sedation is responsiveness to verbal command/light tactile stimuli, as lack of responsiveness means that the patient is going into deep sedation. The level of sedation monitoring must begin before sedation is administered and must continue throughout the procedure and recovery time before the facility is discharged [15]. As patients can respond to a standard dose or medication in an unpredictable manner, and as patients can drift in and out of different levels of sedation, monitoring of responsiveness should be monitored closely and assessed frequently. e.g. the Wilson sedation scale or the UMSS (University of Michigan Sedation Scale). It is proposed that the UMSS is used by sedation practitioners because the rating system matches the sedation levels on the scale of sedation. The importance of the electroencephalogram monitors processed, i.e. bispectral index (BIS) sedation monitoring outside the operating theater, is debatable. BIS might have a role during deep sedation and anesthesia.

3. **Pain and discomfort:** In cases where patients are unable to respond verbally due to the requirements of the procedure, e.g. dental work or head and neck operations, a pain or discomfort signaling device should be established before the sedation starts. This helps patients to prove whether they have pain or discomfort, for example, with thumbs up or thumbs down.

4. **Patency of airways:** Relaxation of the jaw and unintended mouth opening are early indicators of a deepening level of sedation. Noises produced during inspiration or expiration and or snoring suggest a partially blocked upper airway and should be rectified through head and neck repositioning and/or titration of sedation.

5. **Breathing and ventilation:** Throughout the duration of the operation, the breathing rhythm and movement of the chest and abdomen must be observed. Chest movements are expected to be rhythmic. Paradoxical respiration, rib retraction, the use of accessory muscles, and tracheal pull are all symptoms to look out for, all of which can suggest airway obstruction. The respiratory rate should be reported intermittently, except when using a capnograph, where it is constantly displayed. Capnography measures the end-tidal concentration of carbon dioxide, which is considered to be a more sensitive alveolar hypoventilation sensor than pulse oximetry [16, 17].

Patients undergoing PSA tolerate capnography applied via a nasal cannula, side-stream examination and transcutaneous approaches. Capnography is not compulsory for mild sedation, but is strongly advised in patients with fragile ASA II, elderly, obese, obstructive sleep apnea patients, and patients with respiratory problems such as chronic obstructive pulmonary disease (COPD) Nevertheless, Capnography can never replace ventilation/respiration clinical monitoring. If capnography is unavailable, use of a precordial stethoscope may be helpful.

6. **Heart Rhythm and Rate:** For most levels of sedation, the pulse rate, as recorded by pulse oximetry, should be enough. Electrocardiography (ECG) is not necessary in moderate sedation, where regular verbal communication with

the patient is established. However, when using advanced sedation procedures, an ECG is recommended for extended sedation or in delicate ASA II patients, patients with underlying cardiovascular disease and the elderly.

7. **Non-invasive (NIBP) blood pressure.** NIBP must be monitored at all sedation stages.

7. Post-sedation care

Patient is continued to be monitored in the recovery area. Vital signs (blood pressure, heart rate, respiratory rate, oxygen saturation), level of consciousness and level of pain must be monitored and recorded at regular intervals. The recovery area must be staffed with a skilled healthcare professional who certified with at least basic life support. The staff to patient ratio should not exceed two patients to one nurse.

7.1 Scoring systems for discharge

Discharge scoring systems may be used shortly before discharge to identify and record the psychological status of a patient. Modified Aldrete Scoring System (**Table 4**) is widely used to assess when patients from the post-anesthetic care unit are ready for discharge. Patients must score 9 out of 10 before discharge from the recovery room. In addition, the patient must be assisted by a responsible person at home and there must be no complications from surgery, such as bleeding or vomiting. It is no longer important to ensure that the patient is able to take fluids orally, or that before discharge at home, he or she has passed urine. However, if not able to move urine within 6–8 hours of discharge from the sedation unit, the patient must be instructed to contact the responsible practitioner.

Category	Description of Status	Aldrete Score
Respirations	Breathes, coughs freely	2
	Dyspnea	1
	Apnea	0
O2 Saturation	O2 Saturation > 92% on Room Air Supplemental oxygen with O2	2
	Sat > 90%	1
	O2 Saturation < 90% on O2	0
Circulation	BP +/− 20% pre-op value	2
	BP +/− 20–50% pre-op value	1
	BP +/− 50% pre-op value	0
LOC	Awake & oriented	2
	Wakens with stimulation	1
	Not responding	0
Movement	Moves 4 limbs on own	2
	Moves 2 limbs on own	1
	Moves 0 limbs on own	0

Table 4.
Modified Aldrete discharge scoring system (Total *a score of 10 was required for discharge from the endoscopy/ recovery room.*

8. Medications used in GI endoscopy

There is still no perfect medication available for PSA and the combinations of two or more group of agents such as benzodiazepines, opioids, intravenous anesthetics inhalational anesthetics and topical anesthesia is commonly used (**Table 5**). Drug combinations works synergistically which reduces the doses of sedative agents and its side effects. Combination of opioid and sedation is most commonly used regimen. Sedative agents should be titrated to effect in divided doses and the amount of incremental doses should not exceed the maximum recommended doses. In the absence of a weight-related dosage (i.e., mg/kg) for drug doses, the dose for a 'normal' patient weighing 70 kg must be considered to be the dose.

Some anesthesiologist societies advise that general anesthetic inductors (propofol, ketamine, etomidate, dexmedetomidine) and short-acting opioids (fentanyl, alfentanil, sufentanil, remifentanil) should be used only by physicians who have

Medication	dosage	Analgesic effect	Onset	Duration	Side effects
Midazolam	Bolus for deep sedation: 0.1–0.4 mg/kg Bolus for moderate sedation: 0.01–0.1 mg/kg	—	1–5 min	<2 h	Paradoxical excitement (occasionally), hypotension, bradypnea
Propofol	Bolus for deep sedation: 1–2.5 mg/kg Infusion for moderate sedation: 25–100 µg/kg/min	—	<1 min	5–10 min	Hypotension, bradypnea/apnea
Dexmedetomidine	Bolus for deep sedation: 1 µg/kg over 10 min Infusion for moderate sedation: 0.2–0.7 µg/kg/h	++	10–15 min	~30 min	Biphasic hemodynamic effect: bolus administration has been associated with hypertension
Remifentanil	Infusion for moderate sedation: 0.05–2 µg/kg/min	+++	<1 min	5–10 min	Hypotension, bradypnea/apnea, bradycardia
Etomidate	Bolus for deep sedation: 0.2–0.5 mg/kg	—	<1 min	3–5 min	Adrenocortical dysfunction, especially in continuous IV administration
Ketamine	Bolus for deep sedation: 0.5–2 mg/kg Bolus for moderate sedation: 0.2–0.8 mg/kg Infusion for moderate sedation: 10–20 µg/kg/min	++	<1 min	12–25 min	Dissociative hallucination, increased ICP and IOP, tachycardia, and hypertension

ICP, intracranial pressure; IOP, intraocular pressure; IV, intravenous.
Moderate sedation (conscious sedation): purposeful response to verbal commands and intact airway and cardiopulmonary functions; deep sedation: response to painful stimulation and requirement of assistance for proper ventilation and airway patency.

Table 5.
Summary of sedation drugs commonly used.

been specifically trained in anesthesia or intensive care medicine, or by experienced sedation professionals who have at least advanced life support certification and specialized in unique advanced sedation procedures with anesthetic expertise.

Benzodiazepines (e.g. midazolam, diazepam, flunitrazepam, lorazepam or temazepam) and dexmedetomidine are included as procedural sedative drugs. Midazolam is the most widely employed benzodiazepine [18].

Pharyngeal aerosol spray of local anesthetics such as lidocaine, benzocaine may be considered to suppress gag reflex, decrease the dose of sedatives, and facilitate insertion of endoscope. Their effect may last up to an hour.

Benzocaine may cause methemoglobinemia and should be avoided in patients with a previous history of methemoglobinemia or known glucose-6-phosphate dehydrogenase deficiency.

9. Complications of sedation

Sedation-related gastrointestinal endoscopy complications are generally transient and of a mild degree. Nevertheless, when occur, may lead to significant morbidity and occasional mortality especially with moderate and deep sedation. Patient age, comorbidity, as well as type of sedation agent, the dose and route of administration are the most important risk factors of these complications. Serious complications can be avoided by proper pre-operative evaluation, preparation, appropriate monitoring and post-operative management. In addition, skilled treating physicians should be aware, and prepared to treat these complications. Sedation- related endoscopy complications can be divided into cardiovascular, respiratory, gastrointestinal and allergic reactions [19].

9.1 Cardiovascular related complications

Cardiopulmonary related represent 50% of serious sedation related complications and 50% of sedation related deaths in gastrointestinal procedures. Commonly, it occurs in elderly group of patients or secondary to over sedation. Cardiovascular related complications include:

9.1.1 Hypotension

Defined as systolic blood pressure less than 90 mmHg. Generally, systolic blood pressure more than 90 mmHg should maintain mean adequate arterial blood pressure to perfuse all vital organs, BP less than 90 should be treated. Benzodiazepine or opioid a lone rarely causes hypotension. However, combination of both or sedation with propofol, vasovagal attacks and hypovolemia are the most common causes of hypotension [19].

9.1.2 Hypertension

Defined as systolic blood pressure more than 160 mmHg, it is usually secondary to anxiety, pain, intubation and endoscopy.

9.1.3 Cardiac arrythmias

They are commonly observed during gastro-endoscopy. Fortunately, most of arrythmias are benign. Vasovagal attacks, pain and hypovolemia are the most common causes of arrythmia. Opioid and buscopan are associated with bradycardia [15, 19].

9.1.4 Myocardial infarction (MI)

It may occur during endoscopy or within few days post endoscopy. It is commonly reported in patients with history of ischemic heart disease. Hypertension, sever hypotension, tachycardia, pain and anxiety are the leading cause of myocardial ischemia and anginal attacks. The following steps should be considered to treat and prevent perioperative MI and anginal attacks:

1. Pre-oxygentation of high risk patients and continues oxygen supplementation through the procedure.

2. Continue antihypertensive and antianginal medications up to the time of endoscopy.

3. Discontinue the intervention, oxygen supplementation, sublingual nitroglycerine should be considered if angina developed during the endoscopy.

4. 12 lead ECG and request cardiac enzymes if angina or MI are suspected [15, 19].

9.2 Respiratory -related complications

9.2.1 Respiratory depression

Both benzodiazepine and opioids may cause respiratory depression by blocking their receptors in brain and brainstem which may lead to hypoxia and CO_2 retention. Therefore, continues capnography monitoring is extremely important during endoscopic procedures. Drop in oxygen saturation on pulse oximetry is a late sign of respiratory depression especially if patients on supplemental oxygen. Patient stimulation and reversing the sedative agents should be considered to treat respiratory depression. Naloxone (1–2 mcg/kg intravenous) reverses both analgesic and respiratory depressant effect of the opioids, the dose can be repeated every 3 minutes with maximum dose 0.1 mg/kg. Naloxone has short half life (60–90 minutes), therefore patients should be observed at least for 2 hours after administration of naloxone to guarantee that re-sedation does not occur. Flumazenil (0.01 mg/Kg I.V) is a benzodiazepine antidote and useful to reverse both sedative and respiratory depressant effect of benzodiazepine. The half life of flumazenil is 40–80 minutes, therefore patients should be monitored for 2 hours after administration of flumazenil to ensure re-sedation does not occur [19–21].

9.2.2 Air way obstruction

Laryngospasm and bronchospasm are the most common cause of airway obstruction.

9.2.3 Pulmonary aspiration

Pulmonary aspiration of gastric contents during the gastro-intestinal endoscopic procedures are very common. It may lead to pneumonia and death. Over-sedation, gastro-intestinal bleeding, intestinal obstruction, elderly, and hepatic encephalopathy are the risk factors of pulmonary aspiration. Cough, cyanosis and respiratory distress are the early signs of pulmonary aspiration. If the aspiration is suspected, the procedure should be suspended, head down tilt, left lateral positioning, suctioning of the fluid from the airway, encouraging patient and chest x ray should be considered [19].

9.3 Allergic reaction

The wide spectrum of allergic reactions may occur during sedation procedures, it ranges from minor local reaction to life threatening anaphylactic reactions. However, severe allergic reactions during sedation is rare. Diagnosis of anaphylactic reactions under anesthesia is not always easy. Treating physician should immediately stop of most likely precipitating agent, administer adrenaline 0.5 mg intramuscular (IM), secure the airway, administer hydrocortisone, antihistamine as well as IV fluid resuscitation [19].

9.4 Nausea and vomiting

Over-distension of the stomach and colon may induce nausea and vomiting after gastro-intestinal endoscopy. Furthermore, nausea and vomiting are common side effect of opioid agents. Anti -emetic agents such as ondansetron and metoclopramide might be considered to treat sever cases [19, 22].

9.5 Paradoxical reactions

Paradoxical reactions are commonly observed with benzodiazepines especially midazolam and diazepam, it is characterized by agitation, talkativeness, disorientation, combativeness and tachycardia. Flumazenil is very effective in management of these reactions [19, 23, 24].

10. Conclusion

Gastro-intestinal endoscopy is an extremely important diagnostic and therapeutic intervention of gastro-intestinal diseases. Sedation is usually required to alleviate considerable amount of anxiety, discomfort and pain which make the procedure unsafe, complicated and refusal of follow up procedures. Safety of endoscopic procedures under sedation needs awareness of especial needs of the patients. Combination of benzodiazepine and opioid is the most commonly used regimen in gastro-intestinal endoscopy. Though, the gastro-intestinal endoscopy is considered as minimally invasive surgery and sedation for these procedures is generally safe, life threatening sedation related complications may occur easily even in the healthy patients. Pre-procedural risk assessment, preparation, and perioperative as well as post-operative monitoring is mandatory to reduce sedation related complications. Furthermore, properly trained staff and emergency equipment should be available during procedure.

Author details

Moad Ali M. Ehfeda[1*], Adel Ganaw[1], Sohel Mohamed Gamal Ahmed[1], Arshad Chanda[1], Zia Mahood[1], Salem Jabira[2], Hossam Algallie[1], Ahmad H.M. Almaqadma[2], Mahmud M.A. Ben Masoud[2], Ali O. Mohamed Bel Khair[1] and Qazi Zeeshan[1]

1 Department of Anaesthesia, Perioperative Medicine and Critical Care; Hamad Medical Corporation, Doha, Qatar

2 Critical Care Department, Al-Wakra Hospital; Hamad Medical Corporation, Doha, Qatar

*Address all correspondence to: mehfeda@hamad.qa

References

[1] American Society of Anesthesiologists: Continuum of Depth of Sedation: Definition of General Anesthesia and Levels of Sedation/ Analgesia. Approved by ASA House of Delegates on October 13, 1999 and last amended on October 23, 2019. Available at: https://www.asahq.org/standards-and-guidelines/continuum-of-depth-of-sedation-definition-of-general-anesthesia-and-levels-of-sedationanalgesia.

[2] White PF, Ham J, Way WL, Trevor AJ. Pharmacology of ketamine isomers in surgical patients. Anesthesiology. 1980;52:231-9

[3] Tobias JD, Leder M. Procedural sedation: A review of sedative agents, monitoring, and management of complications. Saudi J Anaesth. 2011;5(4):395-410. doi:10.4103/1658-354X.87270

[4] Iyer et al. Mallampati Scores During Pediatric Procedural Sedation and Analgesia. Western Journal of Emergency Medicine. March 2018;19(2). DOI: 10.5811/westjem.2017.11.35913

[5] Reed MJ, Dunn MJ, McKeown DW: Can an airway assessment score predict difficulty at intubation in the emergency department? Emergency Medicine Journal. 2005;22:99-102. https://doi.org/10.1136/emj.2003.008771.

[6] Faramarzi E, Soleimanpour H, Khan ZH, Mahmoodpoor A, Sanaie S. Upper lip bite test for prediction of difficult airway: A systematic review. Pak J Med Sci. 2018;34(4):1019-1023. https://doi.org/10.12669/pjms.344.15364.

[7] ASA Physical Status Classification System. American Society of Anesthesiologists. Archived from the original on 2010-10-08. Available at: https://www.asahq.org/standards-and-guidelines/asa-physical-status-classification-system.

[8] Sharmeen Lotia, MBBS MRCP FRCA, Mark C. Bellamy, MBBS MA FRCA, Anaesthesia and morbid obesity, *Continuing Education in Anaesthesia Critical Care & Pain*, Volume 8, Issue 5, October 2008, Pages 151-156, https://doi.org/10.1093/bjaceaccp/mkn030

[9] Tham TCK, Vandervoort J, Wong RCK, et al. Safety of ERCP during pregnancy. Am J Gastroenterol 2003;987:308-11.

[10] Tang SJ, Mayo MJ, Rodriguez-Frias E, et al. Safety and utility of ERCP during pregnancy. Gastrointest Endosc 2009;69:453-61.

[11] Oh SH. Sedation in Pediatric Esophagogastroduodenoscopy. Clin Endosc. 2018 Mar;51(2):120-128. doi: 10.5946/ce.2018.028. Epub 2018 Mar 30. PMID: 29618173; PMCID: PMC5903085.

[12] American Society of Anesthesiologists Practice guidelines for preoperative fasting and the use of pharmacologic agents to reduce the risk of pulmonary aspiration: An updated report. *Anesthesiology* 126.3 (2017): 376-393

[13] Academy of Medical Royal Colleges. Safe sedation practice for healthcare procedures. Standard and Guidance. October 2013. Available at: https://www.aomrc.org.uk/wp-content/uploads/2016/05/Safe_Sedation_Practice_1213.pdf.

[14] C. G. Sheahan, D. M. Mathews, Monitoring and delivery of sedation, BJA: British Journal of Anaesthesia, Volume 113, Issue suppl_2, December 2014, Pages ii37 ii47, https://doi.org/10.1093/bja/aeu378

[15] Casabianca AB, Becker DE. Cardiovascular monitoring: physiological and technical considerations. Anesth Prog 2009; 56: 53-59; quiz 60 [PMID: 19642720 DOI: 10.2344/0003-3006- 56.2.53].

[16] Waugh JB, Epps CA, Khodneva YA. Capnography enhances surveillance of respiratory events during procedural sedation: a meta-analysis. J Clin Anesth. 2011;23:189-196. https://doi.org/10.1016/j.jclinane.2010.08.012.

[17] Hinkelbein J, Lamperti M, Akeson J, et al. European Society of Anaesthesiology and European Board of Anaesthesiology guidelines for procedural sedation and analgesia in adults. European Journal of Anaesthesiology (EJA). 2018;35(1): 6-24. https://doi.org/10.1097/EJA.0000000000000683.

[18] Jo YY, Kwak HJ. Sedation Strategies for Procedures Outside the Operating Room. Yonsei Med J. 2019 Jun;60(6):491-499. https://doi.org/10.3349/ymj.2019.60.6.491

[19] Somchai Amornyotin. Sedation-related complications in gastrointestinal endoscopy. World J Gastrointest Endosc 2013 November 16; 5(11): 527-533 ISSN 1948-5190. doi:10.4253/wjge.v5.i11.527

[20] British Society of Gastroenterology. Guidelines in Gastro- enterology: Complications of gastrointestinal endoscopy. Available from: http://www.bsg.org.uk/pdf_word_docs/complications.pdf

[21] Amornyotin S. Sedation and monitoring for gastrointestinal endoscopy. World J Gastrointest Endosc 2013; 5: 47-55 [PMID: 23424050 DOI: 10.4253/wjge.v5.i2.47]

[22] Zhang D, Shen Z, You J, Zhu X, Tang QF. Effect of ondanse- tron in preventing postoperative nausea and vomiting under different conditions of general anesthesia: a preliminary, randomized, controlled study. Ups J Med Sci 2013; 118: 87-90 [PMID: 23441598 DOI: 10.3109/03009734.2013.768315]

[23] Robin C, Trieger N. Paradoxical reactions to benzodiazepines in intravenous sedation: a report of 2 cases and review of the literature. Anesth Prog 2002; 49: 128-132 [PMID: 12779114]

[24] Sidhu R, et al. Deep sedation and anaesthesia in complex gastrointestinal endoscopy: a joint position statement endorsed by the British Society of Gastroenterology (BSG), Joint Advisory Group (JAG) and Royal College of Anaesthetists (RCoA) . Frontline Gastroenterology. BMJ. 2019;10:141-147. doi:10.1136/flgastro-2018-101145